# BEAUTIFULLY
# Brave

An unconventional guide
to owning your worth,
cultivating self-love,
and standing in your power

## SARAH PENDRICK

*Founder of* **GIRLTALK**

ROCK
POINT

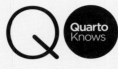

Inspiring | Educating | Creating | Entertaining

Brimming with creative inspiration, how-to projects, and useful information to enrich your everyday life, Quarto Knows is a favorite destination for those pursuing their interests and passions. Visit our site and dig deeper with our books into your area of interest: Quarto Creates, Quarto Cooks, Quarto Homes, Quarto Lives, Quarto Drives, Quarto Explores, Quarto Gifts, or Quarto Kids.

First published in 2021 by Rock Point, an imprint of The Quarto Group,
142 West 36th Street, 4th Floor, New York, NY 10018, USA
T (212) 779-4972  F (212) 779-6058  www.QuartoKnows.com

Rock Point titles are also available at discount for retail, wholesale, promotional, and bulk purchase. For details, contact the Special Sales Manager by email at specialsales@quarto.com or by mail at The Quarto Group, Attn: Special Sales Manager, 100 Cummings Center Suite 265D, Beverly, MA 01915 USA.

10 9 8 7 6 5 4 3 2 1

ISBN: 978-1-63106-748-8

Library of Congress Cataloging-in-Publication Data

Names: Pendrick, Sarah, author.
Title: Beautifully brave : an unconventional guide to owning your worth, cultivating self-love, and standing in your power / Sarah Pendrick.
Description: New York : Rock Point, [2021] | Includes bibliographical references. | Summary: "With Beautifully Brave, foster your inner light through authentic self-love exercises and practices that are easy to use in the real world"-- Provided by publisher.
Identifiers: LCCN 2020054740 (print) | LCCN 2020054741 (ebook) | ISBN 9781631067488 (hardcover) | ISBN 9780760370148 (ebook)
Subjects: LCSH: Self-esteem. | Self-esteem in women. | Self-realization. | Self-realization in women.
Classification: LCC BF697.5.S46 P46 2021  (print) | LCC BF697.5.S46 (ebook) | DDC 158.1--dc23
LC record available at https://lccn.loc.gov/2020054740
LC ebook record available at https://lccn.loc.gov/2020054741

Publisher: Rage Kindelsperger
Creative Director: Laura Drew
Managing Editor: Cara Donaldson
Project Editor: Keyla Pizarro-Hernández
Cover and Interior Design: Evelin Kasikov

Printed in China

*This book is dedicated to you: thank you for showing up for yourself and the world. Thank you for bravely choosing to own who you are by boldly stepping into your deepest love for yourself so that you can show up and make the world a better place. For you are truly beautifully brave.*

# I AM IN THE RIGHT PLACE

# *Introduction*

# WELCOME TO BEING FULLY IN LOVE, WITH YOURSELF

**THE LOVE YOU HAVE** for yourself has the power to heal the world or the power to destroy it. That is how much you matter; that is how much the amount of deep soul searching, unconditional, big love you have for yourself matters.

The reason that the amount of love you have for yourself and the way you express that love matters is because it impacts everything around you. Not only does the love for yourself influence your decisions, your worth, your confidence, and your feelings, but it also impacts the way you live your life and the way you treat others.

We are made of love. We are born of love. Inside every single one of our souls is a desire to love and be loved. If you don't love yourself, you will never be happy. Your love is always there; it's up to you to find it, develop it, and stay committed to being in a relationship with it.

Throughout this book, you will discover, deepen, and reawaken the biggest love of your life (*yourself*) within you. You will be able to share that divine and fierce power with the world and with the people you care about.

In each chapter, you will find a mantra that you can repeat to yourself and several love notes for you to carry with you as you read along. Carry these mantras and love notes with you as little reminders to be kind and loving to yourself. Whenever you are in a moment of need, place your hand on your heart or on your shoulder, and say aloud the words.

Practice creating and repeating compassionate words to yourself every day and come back to this tool any time you need to, to bring yourself back to you and ground yourself back into what is true.

## WHY SHOULD YOU LISTEN TO ME, ANYWAY?

**I KNOW WHOLEHEARTEDLY** within my soul that my purpose here on this earth is to provide support for other women, to give them the support they need to blossom to their fullest potential, and to continue to do that for myself so that I can feel that connection to what's true. When I say what's true, which you will hear me refer to many times, I mean our highest level of being, our fullest expression, our truth.

I didn't always love myself unconditionally growing up. I came into the world as a bright, loud, beautiful young child, completely free and expressive. I wanted to know everything, and I wanted to sing at the top of my lungs. In my experience, I noticed some of my family being uncomfortable with that. I was constantly told that girls shouldn't be like this, girls should be quiet—I was always too loud, too big, and "too much."

Between growing up in a home where I wasn't necessarily encouraged to strive for big dreams—or when I did try to follow my dreams, I was made to feel like I wasn't enough or told I was doing it wrong—and being bullied at school, I struggled a lot with self-esteem. I was always being told by people outside of my home that I thought I was too good for them, that I looked down on them. At home, I was experiencing trauma that made me feel as if I wasn't good enough. It was a crazy set of mixed messages. I didn't know how to handle the disconnect, and so the only way I knew how to exist was to make myself as small as possible. At the time, I wasn't living in my truth.

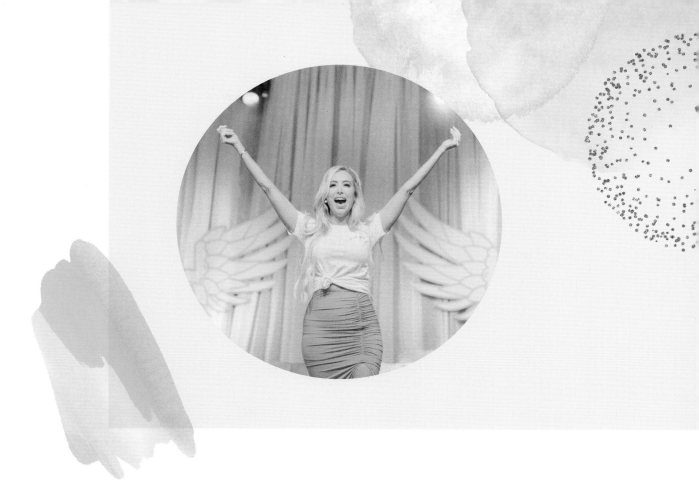

And then, in 2011, after finally being done with allowing judgments and negative projections stop me from pursuing my dreams, I decided to leave my home in Tennessee and move to California. I made the decision after many failed attempts at trying to achieve various goals, losing my dog—who had gotten me through my parents' divorce—and one too many times not taking a risk. I had no plan, no money, and no job. I am a huge believer that when you get a message, that calling in your body that feels like a truth bomb (even when it's feeling insane and you have no idea how it's going to play out), your only job is to follow it: this fearless trust is part of being beautifully brave.

After moving to California, I worked my way into marketing and PR by doing event planning and branding, and discovered that this was something I was good at. I began to open up again, to get big again . . . to get *loud* again—to become me again before anyone else told me what to be or not to be. Before anyone else violated my safety. I remembered days as a child spent holding my teddy bear and speaking my truth to him, telling him all about my feelings and my dreams. I remembered throwing myself into the pool while pretending to be Juliet from *Romeo and Juliet* and creating the biggest splash possible.

I wanted to be a performer. I wanted to be *seen*. And slowly, the space I could create for myself, the role I could play in the world, began to emerge. I could be a performer by sharing my gifts on stage through speaking, facilitating, singing, and creating experiences at my events for audiences while also being an activist, expressing myself and helping others at the same time. And it all started because I followed the message that I received about taking the big risk to move out of state. Even though the move made absolutely no sense and I had absolutely no plan, the minute I trusted myself, I gave myself permission to start to come home to me.

When you begin to live in alignment with your truth, all corners of your life become magical. Three months after moving to LA, I met my husband Josh, my soulmate. The next time I would get another "call" to what was meant for me was when I met him. Our relationship has been a huge part of my growth because I battled with my true knowing, which was that he was meant to be a healing part of my life and my inner child, who was scared to trust, who had been hurt, who had been sexually assaulted, and who had been violated.

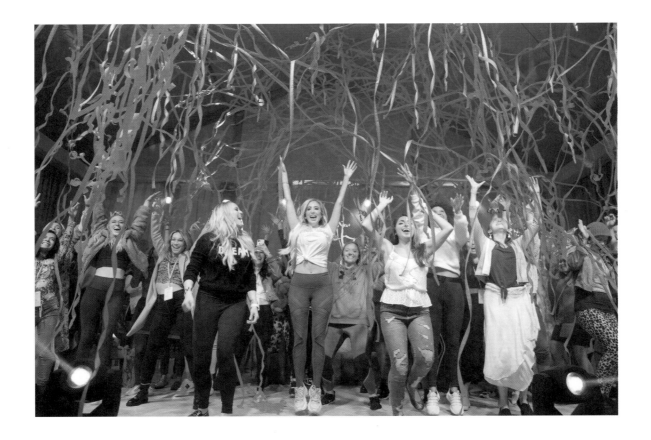

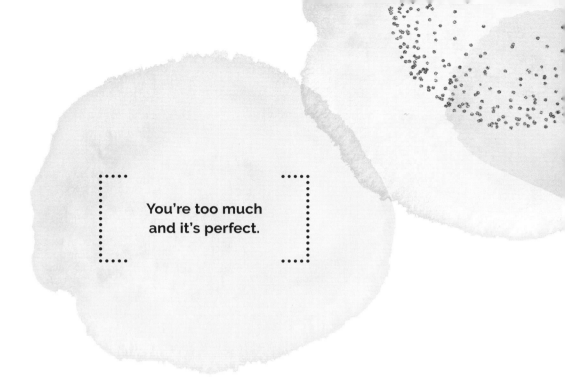

**You're too much
and it's perfect.**

I needed to do some inner healing in order to let this new person into my life and to learn to trust him. My truth chose him, and he turned out to be the man I trust more than anyone I have ever known, the man who showed me that I didn't have to do it all by myself, that I could let go, and be free. The journey of bravery was worth every minute.

When I was growing up, my light was dimmed. I was encouraged to be silent, to conform to outmoded gender roles. But my core belief system from the time I was very young was that women are meant to be "too much." Too much is *exactly* what we should be! Because being myself was impossible in the environment in which I grew up, I set out to create it for myself, and for others.

After a four-year journey of beautifully embracing bravery to become the real me, in 2016, I started my company, a nonprofit called GirlTalk Network. I traveled around the country speaking to women, particularly young women in college, working to support them in their growth and their loudness. And then, over time, GirlTalk grew to become what it is today: a safe space for women of all generations, a place where they can be radically expressive in all of their fullness. A place where women can connect and embrace the tools to live out their wildest and most successful dreams, a place where their dreams manifest into reality.

I met, made friends with, and loved so many incredible women through GirlTalk. I learned something amazing, something that helped me heal and become the "too much" version of myself that I embody with so much joy today: we cannot truly be ourselves unless we love ourselves. Self-love is the rocket fuel that will not only help us fly, but also soar through the stars and journey to places we never believed were possible.

Personal growth and self-development were always a priority for me, but I didn't really know what "self-love" meant for an incredibly long time. In full transparency, I was living in complete survival mode, always five steps ahead so I could stay safe. I was doing the best I could, always searching for answers, yet never finding them. Why? Because, I came to realize later, the thing I needed most was the space to hear my soul. Between doing my own inner work in therapy and being in a program for Masters in Psychology, I slowly began to realize that I was navigating my way to self-love. I never gave up and kept searching for my truth, and without even realizing it, I became an expert in self-love work.

When I decided to move to Los Angeles, everyone told me not to do it. They said I'd be "a little fish in a big pond," doomed to fail, but going there, and succeeding, gave me confidence, which is one of the first steps to self-love! I went from forcing myself to stay quiet to fully living in expression of my bold self. I went from living alone in my heart to feeling filled with love by not only myself, but also by those around me. I went from not knowing how to pay my rent to having a six- and then seven-figure business. My business has allowed me to take a stand for my clients. When they are faced with naysayers, like I was, people who want to protect them but are, in fact, standing in their way, I am someone who believes in them. I believe in their big dreams, in the things they want to create and be in this world. They are not alone.

This book is my way of standing up for *you*. It is a map for your journey of self-work and the continued journey that it will be. Let it guide you along your way.

And so, the following is my love letter to you.

*You are worthy of a big life. You are worthy of happiness. You are worthy of feeling joy and appreciation for yourself and your life every single day. You are meant to be here to experience whatever it is that you desire. You deserve to feel alive, free, and loved. You deserve to have that love from everyone you meet, but most importantly, you deserve to have that love from yourself. It does not matter how old you are or how "young" you are: don't give up on yourself no matter what. Decide today that you are worthy, and decide today to give yourself whatever you need to live the rest of your life experiencing and creating the life you once dreamed of.*

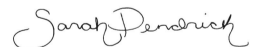

# I AM WORTH IT

# *Chapter 1*

# SELF-LOVE MYTHS

## TRUE SELF-LOVE
## HOLDS YOUR POWER

**WHAT *IS* SELF-LOVE** anyway? We hear the message again and again: "You just don't love yourself enough." What does that even mean?

Self-love is sometimes thrown around like a trending hashtag, like something you do once or on an occasion. If you search the hashtag #selflove online, you'll find millions of pictures that have little to do with the actual true love of the self. If millions of people really loved themselves whole, all the way in, through the ups and downs, and committed to expressing that love publicly in all that they do, then the world would look like a much different place. We aren't there yet. But I believe it's possible, and I believe it starts with you.

Self-love is your commitment to loving yourself no matter what. You will always be on a journey of loving yourself. It is something you continue to redo and undo as you evolve and have different experiences in your life. It's the biggest commitment you will ever make, and despite millions of trending hashtags, it's one of the hardest journeys for people to master. I wish I could tell you that you crack the code and—ta da! That's it, you love yourself! But here's the thing: that love is inside of you. You just have to say *yes*. You will always be evolving in your love for yourself and your connection to you. That doesn't mean that it's hard to do—it's actually really easy! But it takes constant practice because you have a bunch of outside sources messing with you. That is the real hard part. And isn't loving yourself worth it?

The relationship we have with ourselves is often the relationship that we neglect the most . . . and yet, it is the one thing that will have the most impact on those around us. Your self-love will have a positive impact on your children, business partners, friends, family, romantic partners, and anyone who comes in contact with you. It's like a rolling snowball of love, gathering everyone up into its embrace. On the flip side, *not* expressing love for yourself has the power to destroy everything in your path. The lack of expression can turn into a toxic avalanche.

The cycle of pain can repeat itself from generation to generation through thoughts, feelings, and outside experiences during pregnancy. For all the moms out there, data has begun to confirm that stress in the womb can actually affect a baby's body temperature and neurobehavioral development. When a woman is pregnant, her stress levels may cause the baby to show signs of depression or irritability once the baby is born. This is why it is so important for pregnant women to be careful of who they surround themselves with. We have all heard how babies get messages through music or books, and even seem to recognize these sounds or their mothers' voices out of the womb. If this is the case, then, of course babies will be able to pick up and hear other things. This also includes picking up on signals about a mother's mental state. Studies have shown that people have been able to link back their feelings of worthiness, fear, or being "not good enough" to their mother's mental state during pregnancy.

Feelings of unworthiness or being "not good enough" can also carry over onto the next generation through childhood experiences and trauma. Imagine the little one who watched her mother on autopilot, going through her day always in survival mode, being a "good" mom on paper but silently leaving parts of herself behind . . . and in leaving herself, she left her ability to express her love at the door. The mother didn't express love for her daughter or even know how to, because she didn't express love for herself either. The daughter grew up missing her mother's love and missing a part of her. The mother may have done her best—but her daughter may be able to do better. By loving herself whole and expressing that love, the daughter can break that cycle. She has the power to heal the both of them, as will you if you break the cycle by giving yourself love.

If you're reading this and you have a similar story or you resonate with this, say these words: "I can break the cycle. I can love myself. My self-love has the power to go two ways in this world. I choose to be the difference no matter where I am in my life, this starts today."

You are often left with two options when you come from a cycle of pain. You can either be so strong that you choose to fall in love with yourself and show yourself that love every day, or you can continue the cycle and destroy what comes next for you. It's never too late to make a new choice, so don't let yourself buy into that story. You can always make a change for the better.

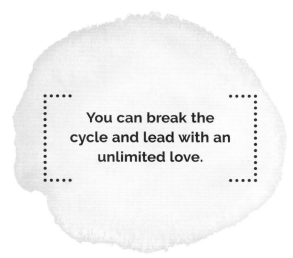

**You can break the cycle and lead with an unlimited love.**

Our expression of self-love is influenced from an early age by our caretakers and the amount of love they show for themselves. You are here to take that power back and bring yourself and those around you back to the truth of falling deeply in love with all parts of you. Falling in love with *you* is the ultimate freedom, and expressing yourself is how you cultivate and deepen it.

## MYTHS ABOUT SELF-LOVE

**SELF-LOVE IS THE** single most important part of yourself. It is the answer to every single thought in your mind, to every worry, to every fear, to everything you ever dreamed of. It is a constant journey, a lifelong commitment, and it never stops. It's also impossible to cultivate if you aren't doing things for yourself to express it. It's not just for those going through a difficult time: it is for every human being on this planet. The deeper you fall more and more in love with yourself, the happier and more connected you will be. This isn't a one-time exercise, you will always be working on loving parts of yourself, for yourself is the single most important relationship you will *ever* have.

There is so much misinformation about what self-love is and isn't. So, let's get all the facts straight, shall we? We'll start by crossing off what self-love *isn't* by smashing four common myths.

## Putting Your Needs First Is Selfish

This myth is a hard one to let go. As mothers, we put our children first. As wives or girlfriends, we put our partners first. As professionals, we put our careers first. As children, we put our parents first. As friends, we put our friends first. Often, *everything and everyone* comes first. It's almost never *us* first.

And why is that? Well, think about it. From a very young age, almost as soon as we are able to be aware of the existence of other people, we are taught to consider their needs. We are told we have to share our toys, our snacks, the attention of the people we love. Of course, this is a necessary part of parenting—after all, we are teaching our children how to exist in a world filled with other people—but it can have some unintended consequences. In learning how to interact in a healthy, loving way with others, we skip over being taught first how to interact with ourselves in a positive way, and the underlying message is that we simply aren't as important as other people.

We aren't taught how to feel into our own needs. We aren't even taught how to discover who we are or feel free to explore who we think we are! We are *told* what we need, whether it's a nap, a snack, or a time-out. Our clothes are chosen for us, our books, our toys, and even our experiences are chosen for us. "You have to share!" "Sit still!" "Don't be too loud!" "Calm down!" These are the messages we receive again and again. This isn't to say it's easy being a parent, after all, we're all doing our best. Societal expectations of children and parenting mean that when your kid is freaking out on the floor of the grocery store, you've got people staring at you and judging you, even though every parent has been there! We are so prone to worrying about what others think, feeling their judgment and our own shame, that we never allow our children the space to feel for themselves.

Now I'm certainly not arguing that a toddler has the decision-making skills necessary to run their own life! But again, the message we receive is that what we want or need—and even who we are—is simply not important. Other people always come first and we better stuff down those feelings or figure out the "right" way to express them. Not to mention, for young girls, we are taught certain gender-confirming behaviors that impact our conditioning. For instance, some things we women often hear growing up are comments like, "Cross your legs when you sit," "Don't play with boys," "Don't wear that, wear this," and the list goes on. Boys also have their own set of conditions, like being told not to cry and to "man up."

Because we are imprinted with limiting beliefs at such a young age, it's so hard to think about our own needs or exactly what we really ought to be doing for ourselves.

**But here's the truth:**
*you are not less important than other people.*

In fact, and bear with me here, because this is going to sound weird—you are *more* important. Your needs come first.

Whoa, what?

I know. It sounds totally wrong.

I'm not saying you are better than anyone else or more important in the greater scheme of things. I'm saying you are more important *to you*. That's all.

I know that doesn't feel right to you, not yet. You've been taught that the opposite is true, and there's a complete unlearning that needs to take place before you can allow yourself to believe and feel that you get to come first and what that really means. Trust me, I'm going to help you get there.

Let's take it one step at a time. Let's look at the ways in which you put yourself last, every day. For example, think of the times when you're asked to go for drinks with friends, and you love them, but you just really want a night in, and you go anyway because your friends want you to. Even when you don't go, what do you tell them? I bet you have come up with a bunch of excuses similar to, "Oh, sorry, I have to work!" Or, "My boyfriend is sick." Why do we do this? It's because we know that our friends—really, everyone—will be much more able to accept the explanation if we say we are putting someone else's needs first, rather than simply saying we don't want to go. But what would happen if we simply said, "I'm going to stay home and take care of myself tonight"? I cannot wait for you to test this out. Believe me, you will soon enough, and you get to take all the important people in your life on that same empowerment journey of love. If they're willing, and if they're not, you'll learn about that, too!

I wish that I could tell you your friends would applaud your healthy choices, but unfortunately that kind of direct self-love and self-care might hit them like a splash of cold water. It's a shock to the system to hear someone put themselves and their needs first like that; after all, our friends went through the same internalization process that made them think that the "right" way to exist in the world is to put other people first. Your friends might not necessarily think you're being selfish, but it would be hard for them to understand, because it's so foreign to us as humans in this society to even consider putting our own needs first.

This is definitely more of an issue for women than it is for men. Even though men, for the most part, get the same messages about putting others first when they are very young, those messages shift as they get older. It is simply more acceptable for a man to say, "I'm going to go to the gym" when the baby needs changing. If a woman were to say that, it would feel wrong, like she's avoiding her responsibilities or not doing her fair share—she would feel like she's placing a burden on her partner.

There are more rules for women in these situations, and more judgment when we break those rules. We judge ourselves, and we judge other women. It's natural, and it happens because we still haven't unlearned these messages about our importance and place in the world. When we see a woman who *has* done this work and is putting herself first, it can be shocking. We are triggered, and we can feel almost angry or envious of her. And that anger comes from a place deep inside, a natural, free place where we know that we should be living with that kind of freedom . . . but we aren't, not yet. We feel a little envious, and we put judgment on this woman to make ourselves feel better because she is doing the very thing that we somewhere inside wish we were doing too.

## SMASH THE MYTH

The first step is always awareness. Now that you know where this idea came from that putting yourself first is selfish, you can start to unlearn it. This will take time—it's not easy to undo years of childhood and cultural imprinting. But with practice it's totally possible. Every time you put yourself first, it will get easier. You'll feel a little less selfish (yes, you will *feel off*, especially at first, but that doesn't mean you *are* wrong), and a little less judgmental of yourself, until eventually it feels aligned and exactly as it should be to put yourself first—which it absolutely is! This is one of the first actions you can take to start unlearning this myth.

As you practice putting yourself first, sit with these questions:

What does "put me first" feel like in my body?

What happens when I do put myself first?

If I can break through these untrue cultural beliefs, how will I live differently?

How will my life and the lives of the people I care about improve if I put myself first?

How will putting myself first impact my kids, my friends, my family, the world?

---

**MYTH #2:**

### You Have to Love Yourself Just as You Are

The idea of loving yourself just as you are sounds so great, right? Isn't that what love is? We all want to be seen and appreciated for who we are. And shouldn't loving yourself work that way, too? Yes . . . but also no. You absolutely should love yourself just as you are, but you can't just leave it there, because your essence, who you are, wants you to evolve and grow. And when you're not, you will feel it.

If we love ourselves just as we are and we don't do anything to improve, learn, or uplevel, then we will never grow and will be suffering inside—humans need growth! Complacency is the worst thing you could do for yourself. Imagine having nothing to strive for, nothing to be proud of, nothing to want out of life. What a stagnant, dull, depressing existence! You would be stuck in a life you aren't happy with. And if you are feeling stuck now or have been before, I love you. I have been down before, and most everyone I know has as well. You aren't and won't be stuck in that negative space. More on this later . . .

We crave growth, and we crave change. Loving ourselves not only means accepting and loving things as they are but also recognizing that we have the power to grow, and that positive shift is a gift we can give ourselves.

Someone once asked me if I'd rather be a failure all the time or a success all the time. The correct answer is neither! Both answers are static. That phrase "all the time" is a trap. Obviously, no one wants to be a failure all the time, that's a given—imagine sitting in that muck! You would be learning from your failures, but chances are, you would also be chasing the need to be "good enough." Choosing success all the time is just as tormenting, because then nothing will ever feel like a true success and there will never be room for growth or transformation.

The place to be is right in the middle, where you're striving, but feeling acceptance about yourself at the same time. Love yourself as you are now, but remember that part of your love for yourself is your desire to do more and achieve more, and then doing something about it.

I have to tell you, this myth hits me pretty hard, and I still struggle with it sometimes. When I was growing up, I liked pretty things. I liked to look good, and I still do! But I remember my dad saying to me, "The people in our family aren't gorgeous." Someone had called me gorgeous, and my dad's comment immediately kept me from feeling the pleasure and joy of receiving that compliment in that moment, and the confidence and sense of gratitude it gave me. What I heard was: "You're not pretty." With that message in mind, loving myself just as I was would have meant loving myself as "not pretty," and simply accepting that as a fact and not doing anything about it. If I'd stayed stuck in that muck, I would have never made the choice to not allow his lack of knowing how to nurture me in that moment to impact my self-esteem.

My dad told me years later that he didn't want me to think that looks were everything or allow people to judge me on how I did or did not look. He wanted to make sure that I didn't think that looks were everything. And they're not, but his comment took a precious moment away from me and left room for an insecurity to form. He was protecting me with his actions colored by his concerns around the importance that society places on appearance.

Where does this myth even come from? Why do we do this?

I think it comes from the same place my dad's comment came from—fear. When we take an attitude of "everything's great just as it is" even when that's not true, we are trying to protect ourselves from disappointment. What if we can't change? What if we can't grow? What if we try and we fail?

I love myself
when I put my needs
first and when I give
myself the space
to grow.

Fear of disappointment stops so many of us from trying. But we can *always* change. There's always a solution. Maybe you need a shift in mind-set or a new outlook. Maybe you need to learn a new skill or take a risk! There's *always* something you can do.

If you look at a part of yourself that you want to change—whether it's your hair, or your job, or your cooking skills, or whatever—and you simply decide not to do anything about it, you're actually stopping yourself from being able to truly love that part of you. Instead, you're settling. Instead of trying to push it away and saying, "Oh, I love this," embrace your "crazy" hair, try new things, own up to hating your job, and get curious about how you can either start loving it or lose it for something better. If you do not explore options or give yourself the permission and opportunity to desire something more, you're holding yourself back and, I hate to say it but, you're just pretending that everything is fine. No matter how hard you try, at some point the truth will always come back around, and then you'll have no choice but to face it head on. Going on with life pretending doesn't work; it always catches up to you, and deep inside, you always know the truth, pretending that you don't, only hurts you more.

Most often, though, we don't even allow ourselves to see the parts of us that aren't what we want them to be. We look away out of fear and pretend they aren't there. Or we focus only on the one thing we don't love, ignoring all the things we do love and ultimately enter into a spiral of negativity shooting us further away from appreciating ourselves. Unless you can love yourself enough to shine a light and really look at what you want to change and why, you will never accept fully. It's simply not possible to love something you're settling for, even when it's a part of you. The key is to explore and face it, once you do that, all the answers will appear.

Let's say you're not happy with your body. If you tell yourself, "It's okay, I'm just going to love it the way it is," then you're not empowering yourself to make choices to give your body healthy foods, to exercise, to support and take care of your body in a way that shows how much you love it and appreciate it. Next time you aren't happy with something, do the work to give it love and care and then see what happens. What matters inside is that you can honestly say with all things that you gave it the attention and love that it deserved. The results will not matter as much as the love that was given, and the only opinion that will matter will become your own. It is also important to note here that when you don't shine a light on things, you shame them, and shaming a part of you is the exact opposite of healing and loving yourself.

At heart, the myth of loving yourself just as you are is completely illogical. Look at it this way: if you've got dry skin, are you supposed to just say, "Yay! I love my dry skin just the way it is!" Or are you allowed to, you know, put on some lotion? If your relationship has problems, are you supposed to just love it the way it is? Or should you and your partner talk about your problems, seek therapy, and try to work it out? You deserve the same amount of care, effort, and help.

> **Loving yourself doesn't mean giving up on yourself! It means caring enough about yourself to put in some work and pushing back against your fears while diving into why those fears are there.**

As I mentioned earlier, I still have trouble with this myth sometimes, and I have to keep practicing overcoming my own fear of disappointment. When you're struggling, ask yourself these questions:

What am I afraid to admit I want to change about myself?

What would it mean to love myself enough to take a risk?

How would my life be different if I allowed myself to grow?

How will my life, and the lives of the people I love, improve if I loved myself and wanted to grow and learn?

I love myself
when I let
myself rise.

## The Self-love Journey Is Only for Those Who Are Having a Tough Time

This is one of my favorite myths because I encounter it in people all the time—people you wouldn't expect to be having any issues with "self-love." I'll meet this incredibly successful woman—she's confident, she's passionate, and she feels like she's absolutely living her best life. And guess what? Turns out, she's not doing the work, the inner work, or expressing love for herself.

The clue is in the phrase "best life." How do you *know* you're living your best life? It might look like it from the outside, and you can be really proud of what you have and what you've accomplished . . . but you don't get to cross your life off like a checkbox on a to-do list. Life doesn't work like that! At least not a truly fulfilled one. When I really get to talking with this successful woman, it turns out she has an even bigger dream, one that she's not allowing herself to pursue because she doesn't believe she's capable of achieving it.

I had a client, Megan, who came to me for business coaching. She sat down in my office with a beautiful smile, a fresh notebook, and an adorable blazer that showed me she was serious. She had recently left a career she hated and wanted to start her own business. She was asking me for all kinds of practical, external advice (and to be honest, most of what I was telling her she already knew), but during every follow-up meeting, she revealed that she hadn't done any of the things we discussed.

As this so often happens, it became clear that she didn't need business coaching, she needed something else, but she never did any of the things we figured out she needed to do to launch her new career. She simply wasn't following through. We moved into personal development coaching. We dug into the inner work necessary to give her the confidence to actually start this business she dreamed of. We traced it back to her recent divorce from a narcissistic husband, to her family, and began to move through the healing process of self-work and self-doubt. At first, she thought all she needed was the business advice; she didn't think that anything else was necessary, but doing the inner work *always* is. And now she has a thriving business, oozes self-confidence, and loves and honors all of herself and what's best for her.

If you truly wanted to go for all your huge desires, you could. Believing in yourself would be a large factor in them happening. You don't wake up every day believing in yourself; life will throw you off, and that is exactly where being in touch with yourself and making your inner work a nonnegotiable come in.

But maybe you're doing pretty well. You've got a good life, you like your job, you like your home, you mostly get to do the things you want to do, and you're feeling pretty good about things. Guess what? You *still* get to nurture yourself because you are better than feeling "pretty good." Imagine what it would feel like to be so in love with you, incredibly connected, and full of joy! Sounds better than feeling pretty good, yes? And I imagine there is something inside you that is calling for more self-expression, for something more. If you are living in complete joy, you're going to pass that joy on to others, and when you pass love on to others, you still get to fill your cup of joy back up again and again.

We can feel shame around this. We think, "Who am I to ask for more? There are so many people struggling, and I have so much. I should feel great! That's just self-indulgent." Hear this now: *loving yourself is never self-indulgent.* Every single person on this planet needs more and more love, no matter how "successful" they are. Each of us may be at a different place in our journey of self-love, but that's exactly what it is—a journey. It is an ever-expanding practice and a never-ending feeling of deep self-compassion that is available to you. Just like a monk working to reach enlightenment, there is always more light to be sought. You will always have more love to give yourself, and you will always need to express it.

Think about self-love like you think about a relationship. Relationships take work, even the very best ones (they are actually the best because of the work!). If you want to cultivate your relationship, you always need to tend to it. The work of a relationship is never done, no matter how well it's going. And the same is true of your relationship with yourself—it's constant practice and giving.

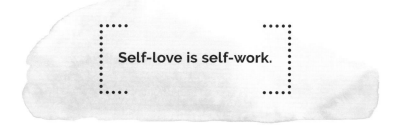

**Self-love is self-work.**

I was recently on a Mastermind Retreat with eight super-powerful, amazing women, all of them with seven-figure businesses. We were working on both our business and our personal growth (because the two always go hand in hand!), and when we all went around and talked about what was standing in our way, preventing us from taking the next steps in our business, it was never something outside of us or something practical.

For each and every one of us, it was some inner block of not feeling good enough or worthy enough to take that next step and reach that next level. I shared my truth, and by listening to the other women, I realized that I wasn't alone, and neither are you. Whether you have a seven-figure business, are not working, or are just entering the workforce, know that you aren't alone in your doubts. But that doesn't mean these doubts have to persist!

I had a similar situation with one client, Trish, in my women's leadership Mastermind, "Together We Empress." She serves an amazing community and was absolutely ready to grow and expand that community, but she also had some doubts holding her back. She was stuck with the idea that she already had reached everyone in her small region. At first, what I was hearing her say was that there wasn't more available to her. She's got a huge following outside of the US, but for some reason, she believed she couldn't succeed in America. She didn't have the confidence in herself to think she could understand and serve people in the US—despite how much she was offering the rest of us in my coaching group, half of whom were living in America and looked to Trish as a huge business inspiration. Even though I could see her so clearly (and so could the rest of my clients—our Mastermind sisters), she needed to do the self-work necessary to grow her belief in herself, to gain the confidence to speak to a broader audience. You can seek outside validation, but until you begin to validate yourself, work through the roots of your self-doubts and limitations, and choose to walk through your fears, you will stay stuck in life.

> **Every single person, no matter where you're at, needs to continue to do the inner work. There's always self-work to do and more love to express.**

This myth can be difficult to break apart because there's a slight kernel of truth to it. When we struggle, that's when we need our self-love practices the most, but we also struggle because we aren't expressing our love for ourselves in the first place. It's an unfortunate vicious cycle, but there's a way out of it. Don't wait until you hit your lowest point to give yourself love. Instead practice, cultivate, and grow your connection with yourself *all the time*, even when things are going great. The best news is, we dive into all the ways you can do that in the chapters ahead.

Ask yourself:

How do I know that I love myself?

In what ways do I show myself love?

How would my life be different if I showed up for myself all the time?

How will my life, and the lives of the people I love, improve if I start to show up bigger, more of myself, and brighter every day?

## Self-care Has Nothing to Do with Self-love

This myth doesn't even make sense! Of *course* self-care is about loving yourself. But once again, this is an instance where the world of social media and trending hashtags have turned something as simple and obvious as self-care into something people look at as a luxury. Self-care has a rep. It's for people who are high maintenance, maybe even spoiled. According to the internet, self-care means getting your nails done, getting a massage, or wearing a cute outfit.

Honestly? This myth is ridiculous.

Just like how you can't drive a car without gas, you can't function fully as who you are without self-care. Period. It's not a luxury; it's a necessity.

In the past, I totally bought into this myth. I started feeling bad about my self-care practice and what I thought it said about me, and I wanted to tear off that "high-maintenance" label. And so, I put a halt on my practice and stopped setting aside time and space for myself. And wow, did that backfire. Before too much time had passed, I began feeling distanced from myself because I wasn't taking care of me or I was so "busy" that I wasn't listening to myself, in this time, I saw how much I needed self-care and the space it creates. It allows me to be close to myself and hear what my heart truly wants.

The more you keep going and going without setting aside time for self-care, the further away you move from yourself . . . and the harder it becomes to get back into alignment.

To be frank, we've got some pretty crazy ideas about what self-care is supposed to look like. Self-care isn't necessarily something that looks good on social media! It's really very simple: it's time that you give yourself to connect with your body, to get an energy boost, to carve out some space just for you. The images that you carry in your mind of what self-care means may not be self-care for you . . . or maybe they are! Listen, maybe your idea of self-care *is* getting a massage or a manicure, and if so, that's fantastic! There's nothing at all wrong with pampering yourself sometimes, or with wanting to look good or feel good. Damn straight that's self-care.

But that's not *all* self-care can be. It can be going out with friends. It can be going on a hike. It can be journaling. It can be going to the gym, or doing yoga, or making soap, or gardening, or taking a nap. I don't know what self-care looks like for you. Nobody does—except you!

I love myself when I do the inner work to show up for myself and take time for self-care.

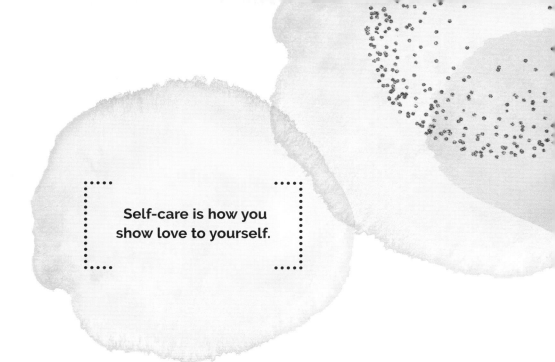

> **Self-care is how you show love to yourself.**

How do you show love to people? You give them things, you provide for them, you do things for them, you tell them how you feel every day. How would you do this for *you*? It may take some internal inquiry to figure out what your version of self-care is, but you'll get there, and we will dive into that on this journey to come.

The most common argument against self-care is that we don't have time for it. Honestly, if I hear one more woman tell me she doesn't have time for self-care, I'm going to shake her (with love, of course!). Don't you *ever* say you don't have time for self-care. This is possibly the most valuable way you could spend your time, so you'd better be setting aside time in your schedule for it!

I get it, you're busy. Maybe you're trying to grow a business, or you have little ones at home. But in the long run, setting aside time for self-care is the best thing you can do for that business or your loved ones. My friend Jenn was working like crazy trying to get her clothing boutique up and running. It was her dream and it made her soul really happy, so she was putting all her time into it. As part of our self-care routine, she and I used to go to Pilates together every week, but she started skipping it. In fact, I hadn't talked to her in weeks until I got a panicked phone call from her. She was completely overwhelmed and hadn't planned well enough. Orders were rolling in and she didn't have time to get them organized, much less packaged and sent out the door. I saw right away what the problem was—she needed an assistant. She was concerned about her bottom line and had instead decided to do everything herself, putting her own needs at the bottom of the priorities list.

In reality, she was actually hurting her bottom line by trying to do it all on her own. Together, Jenn and I figured out a plan of action to handle this crisis, and then quickly got her an amazing assistant. Soon, she was back at Pilates with me and thriving in her business and in her personal health. What she learned in that experience is that setting aside time for herself to breathe and move her body gave her the space to figure out what she could handle and where she needed support. It allowed her to make better decisions for her business because when we are on the go and keeping everything in our head with no space for ourselves we are bound to explode, and the very thing keeping us "so busy" will come tumbling down with us. Can you think back to a time that you've been in this same spot as Jenn? Maybe it's right now.

What could bring you a sense of peace in those moments? For you, maybe it's 10 minutes spent in meditation. Maybe it's snuggling up to your babies and breathing in the scent of their skin. Maybe it's 3 minutes of complete silence (I highly recommend trying this!). Self-care doesn't have to mean hours and hours away from work, or family, or responsibilities. A little definitely goes a long way, and the rewards are incredible. Showing yourself care is showing yourself love and it brings you back to yourself. It also inspires you. Think about it, have you ever gotten huge ideas when you're in the shower or working out? When you give to your mind and body, your soul has a chance to give right back.

> **When you practice self-care that is unique to you, you show yourself how worthy you are to be cherished. You are showing the universe that you will take care of the beautiful person that you are meant to be.**

The thing about this myth is that it's kind of all the myths I mentioned above rolled into one. "Self-care is selfish." "Self-care isn't necessary because I'm fine just as I am." "Self-care is only for when things are going badly, when I really need it." Do any of those phrases sound like the voice in your head?

Self-care is the deliberate practice of activities that "take care" of mental, emotional, and physical health. When you practice self-care, you improve your immune system's function, decrease any feelings of depression or anxiety, and increase your empathy towards others.

Because this myth is wrapped up with all of the others, it can be a hard one to let go. The good news is there's a whole chapter on this later on! But for now, start thinking about what self-care means for you. You can look at society's definition or at your family's definition, and then start paying attention to what makes you feel good and loved. Self-care is part of your love language with yourself—start figuring out how to translate it!

Ask yourself:

**What do I think self-care is supposed to look like?**

**What might self-care really look like for me?**

**How would my life be different if I made time for self-care every day?**

**How will my life, and the lives of the people I love, improve if I practiced real self-care?**

I love myself
when I freely express
it and take care of
my needs.

# 10 WAYS TO DEBUNK SELF-LOVE MYTHS

**1** **Lead with unlimited love.** Break the cycle of pain and take the time to heal the part of you that needs healing. Live a life full of love for yourself and see how the world around you becomes more loving.

**2** **Take your power back.** Be kind to yourself and give yourself love. When we do this, we become free to express ourselves.

**3** **Take the time to unlearn some of the limiting behaviors you were taught to believe in.** What are those behaviors? How have they shaped your life and how can you unlearn them every day? It will take some time to do this, but you will get there.

**4** **Put yourself first.** This will take some time to get used to, but you can do it with some practice. How will you put yourself first today?

**5** **Be open for change and growth.** We should definitely love ourselves, but part of growth happens when we are open to change and constantly evolving. Change involves a lot of risk taking, so take a risk and take action towards the life you want!

**6** **Practice self-love always.** Self-love is not just for when you aren't feeling good or struggling. It's something you practice consistently even when your life feels like it's heading in the right direction.

**7** **Always do the inner work.** Make your inner work a nonnegotiable. When you take the time to look within, you become unstoppable.

**8** **Take time for self-care.** We need to take care of ourselves; self-care is a necessity not a luxury. Don't just practice this when you are having a hard time or stressed at work, do it ALL the time. This way you make sure you are loving yourself every day and giving yourself the space to take care of your needs.

**9** **Figure out what self-care looks like to you.** Self-care is not a one-stop shop and it looks different for everybody. Your self-care may consist of a few minutes of silence or going on a great adventure.

**10** **Know that self-love is a never-ending journey.** Self-love work is something that we continue to do daily. There will be days when it will be hard to express love for yourself, so it is important to continue to practice self-love. By cultivating self-love in our every day we are continuing to break the cycles of pain and trauma and choosing to give ourselves healing.

## Homework: Self-assessment

The most important thing you can give yourself is the power of your own love. Your self-love journey will take some time, and as I've mentioned earlier in this chapter, it will take a lot of unlearning self-love myths to get started with loving yourself. To get started in your own journey, take a serious look at the things that have stopped you from embracing who you are at the core. Think about the ways you have or have not expressed yourself and why that might be. Don't ever let anything stop you from being "loud." You are worthy of the kind of love you want and wish to have. You are more than enough and have the power to change the world.

Here are some quick steps to follow so you can debunk these myths on your own and get through the tough stuff.

**Step 1:** The phrase "smash the myths" is about getting honest with the myths and external opinions you've allowed to control what is and is not acceptable for you. Take a moment and think about how some of the self-love myths have shaped who you are at this moment.

- What myths have I given in to in the past?
- What myths will I stop giving in to?
- In what ways will I stop giving in to these myths?

Make it a habit to check in with yourself daily or weekly on what you have or have not been accepting for yourself. Soon you will start to notice whenever you are falling into the trap of these myths and can then refocus the love back on you.

**Step 2:** Dive into loving yourself and empowering yourself by showing up for you. This could mean starting to say "no" to things that don't serve you or taking some time for self-care during the week.

- How have I been showing up for myself today?
- Where in my life and in what ways have I *not* been showing up for myself?

**Step 3:** It's time to throw out what hasn't been working and figure out what has been working for you. Begin to let go of the things that are not serving you and are draining your energy. Say "yes" to the things that bring that spark of joy into your life. A good way to start is by asking yourself what self-love means for you. Once you figure that out, you'll be able to take actionable steps toward loving you.

- What was I taught about self-love?
- What is my definition of it?
- What have I been doing lately that has been making me happier?
- What am I accepting or doing that may be draining my energy?

**Higher Love Level:** Over the course of each chapter, you may start to notice that your thoughts, viewpoints, and self-concept are transforming and rising in unexpected ways. Keep a journal of your thoughts and bookmark parts that speak to you as you read along. After you are on the other side, come back to this homework assignment, and you may be surprised at what your new answers will be!

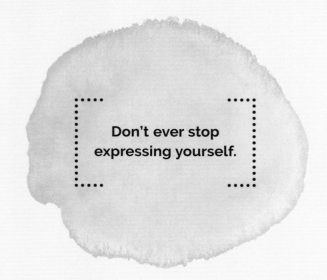

**Don't ever stop expressing yourself.**

# MY STRENGTH IS GREATER THAN MY STRUGGLES

# Chapter 2

# THE SCIENCE
# OF HAPPINESS

**THERE ARE TWO** types of happiness. The first is hedonic happiness. This is the happiness you see in social-media highlights, or the chase of the bad boy or the bad girl. Think of these as a quick hit of dopamine you get when you reach for a certain snack or an unhealthy habit; it is what you see in ads, quick fixes, or shiny objects. It is what you feel in those brief moments of satisfaction or pleasure. It is the type of happiness that is not lasting.

Have you ever wondered why you got that bag you had been obsessing over, or that car, or (insert your dopamine hit here), and realized that lasted about a minute, a day, a week? So, you reach for more, another thing, another object, another quick hit. Trust me, I am all about everyone getting those luxury items, so that is not what I am saying (we will get to this later), but when we leave our happiness only up to those quick fixes, we wake up feeling lost, confused, unhappy, and needing more.

My dear friend Dr. Judy Ho, triple board-certified and licensed clinical and forensic neuropsychologist, media personality, and published author, explained that when you reach for the quick fixes too much, you deny your mind the chance to sit with the uncomfortable feeling, causing you to run away and miss out on the experience of self-reflection. And when you run away from something, it starts to become a fear. But if you decide to experience the negative emotion, you start to confront the fear.

> **When you turn around to face whatever it is that is going on inside you, you are able to build resilience inside yourself.**

When you confront the fear, it gets smaller because you survived it. When you confront negative feelings, you conquer your fear, and you build the knowing that you are able to conquer anything that comes your way. This creates a much stronger and longer-lasting happiness. This leads me to the second type of happiness . . . eudaimonic happiness. This is the type of happiness that is lasting. You receive this through living in your values, accepting your whole self, loving yourself, being mindful, pursuing things that ignite the purpose inside of you, and cultivating positive relationships. You receive this lasting happiness that you receive through self-reflection and well-being. To put it simply, hedonic happiness is created through actions of pleasure and enjoyment, while eudaimonic happiness is achieved through experiences of meaning and purpose. And while it's clear that lasting happiness is key, psychologists have found that people require both types of happiness in order to flourish.

When it comes to happiness, we often get it wrong because we think that happiness means the absence of negative emotions. We think once we are happy, we will never experience pain again. I mean, come on, do we make things more complicated than they have to be or what? Who decided that being happy meant never feeling a negative emotion again? Let's talk about an impossible standard to hold! The surprising thing is, there are some benefits to experiencing pain. A psychological study published by SpringerLink found that experiencing pain can benefit your defense systems, which, in turn, makes you more motivated. Not only that, but it reduces feelings of guilt or self-indulgence. I'm by no means saying to go put yourself in a painful situation, but if you are in one, realize there are benefits to be found.

True happiness is living a life full of meaning, and only you can decide what truly means something to you. When you are pursuing anything that has meaning, there will always be some struggle. It's with that struggle that you either create more fear or you bravely conquer it and build feelings within yourself that create things you can be proud of.

# KNOWING YOUR TOP VALUES
# CULTIVATES LASTING HAPPINESS

**CULTIVATING HAPPINESS IS** about having a meaningful life and creating your own definition of success. Because success is widely talked about in society, let's use "success" right now as an example. The idea that happiness only happens when success happens is where we get the idea of happiness mixed up, because it's really cultivated through the process of living. Everyone has heard the phrase "It's the journey, not the destination." The journey is about the experiences of life, and when you are in pursuit of what really means something to your truest self, and it's something you value, it gives you a sense of deep purpose because you are doing what you love. And when bumps come along the road, which is inevitable, you will strengthen your motivation and resilience because you are doing what makes you feel most authentic. When you are doing what is most authentic to you, you have a strong sense of self and are not as easily influenced by external opinions. And once you get to the destination, you have a deeper sense of well-being, truth, and joy in the entire experience.

Loving yourself is knowing who you are. It's expressing yourself. It's being the unlimited love that you seek to find and finding it inside of you. Your values change as you grow—this is why it's important to constantly check in with them and to know them. You are a multidimensional person, and because part of living is growing, expressing, and expanding, what is meaningful to you will be shifting as you expand. This is a compass, a tool in your purse, guidance that will serve you at all times. These "values" are accessible whenever you need them. A tool to always have with you is knowing what is meaningful to you. When you know this information and you are constantly evolving and checking in with yourself, you have something available to you whenever you feel struggle, disconnection, a low vibration, or negative emotions. Knowing your values will not only make you happier, it will increase your level of confidence because it creates a sense of stability and safety in your life. When you know what you want, it no longer matters what other people want. When you know what is important to you, it doesn't matter what is important to other people over your own desires. In order to have this foundation to turn to, you must know your values.

The word *value* is defined as "something of importance or worth." Do you know what is most important to you in life? Do you know what your values are? Have you ever checked in on this or have you checked in on this lately? You cannot copy someone else's values; they must be your own. Look to yourself to know these and evolve them when needed. This is a way to stand in your power during difficult times and a way to love yourself more deeply.

You may be wondering, how do I know what my values are? Let me give you some steps to follow so that you can begin to dive into your values and what is most meaningful to you while you read through this chapter.

**Follow these steps to figure out what matters to you.**

 Pull out a notebook and begin to write down all the words, feelings, and ideals that you embody or admire. These could be words like family, community, respect, freedom, humor, health, spirituality… you get the idea. Let your mind be open to listing as many words that come into your thoughts as possible.

 Refine this list down to four to five words. Which ones do you resonate with the most? Be mindful of the words that you feel a body response to. This will usually show you what your top values at that moment are and what is important to you at your core.

 Spend time writing what you believe each value means. Your idea of self-expression or community could be vastly different from someone else's, so get clear on what your values are to you so that you can then take them and build your days and life around them.

One of the things that is most valuable to me, something that feels very strong inside of me, is sisterhood. Blame it on having three brothers or maybe because Mother Nature rewards sisterhood and it's a natural place inside of us as women. I know that in order for me to cultivate a higher vibration I have to honor sisterhood—a deep sisterhood, not just some friends that I can call up and chat with. I incorporate this into my world. I have a standard for it. I do not settle and when I feel struggle, I find a way to ignite sisterhood. This is why my work is centered so much around women and it is also what led me through the years to feel connected to myself. When you live in alignment with your values, you will walk closer to your own heart and spirit.

Because sisterhood is deeply meaningful to me, I allow it to happen, and I allow myself to be on this journey.

When you are coming up against something, ask yourself how you can take a quick break and honor one of your values or honor something that has a deep meaning for you. The way you find what makes a difference to you and what is important to you in life is by taking the space to ask yourself what they are. What do you usually take a stand for? What brings you joy that when you do it, you can feel your body fill up with excitement? What do you feel inside your core is important to have in life?

Let's say you value adventure. If this is true, then you know that part of cultivating your high frequency is by having adventure in your life. You can practice having adventure in your life by going outside for 10 minutes, going on a bike ride, running, or hiking. Or if, for example, you feel deep meaning in connection, while you might not be able to go to a party at the drop of a hat, you can practice connecting with others by picking up the phone and talking with a loved one. You could send something to someone, hug someone, or go inward and connect to your inner voice.

**If something is costing you your happiness, it's too expensive. Invest in something else.**

As I spoke with Dr. Judy Ho about the importance of value work, she reminded me that so often people think they must make big moves that they forget the little steps or the little things that matter too. You can also have the same neurochemical influence on your brain in small doses. We spoke about how we have both heard people say, "I was happy for like 10 minutes while doing it, so what?" The thing is, the more you build in little positive moments for yourself, the more your brain will build in this frequency. Dr. Ho said, "The little positive habits are basically the foundation for your life." By doing little things each day that make you happy and honor what you value, you will create higher and higher jolts of this frequency in your brain.

# YOUR THOUGHTS CREATE YOUR REALITY

**NOW IT'S TIME** to take you down the rabbit hole where science and spirituality intertwine. While science is important because it shows us proven facts, there are also things that you cannot and will not ever be able to find an explanation for. That is when faith, knowing, and a little bit of magic come in. These are the things that no one can possibly understand how they happened, or they happened against all odds. Because miracles do happen. And guess what, you can actually attract and be a magnet for them too. Our true nature and our nature as women is to embrace, trust, and be open to these signs and miracles because that is part of our power within, our divine femininity.

But let's start with the science of how your thoughts create your reality. You may have heard this before. Or perhaps you've heard about the law of attraction. I believe it's important to understand the science behind these concepts because otherwise (for some) this all can sound a little "woo woo." Once you understand that the entire universe is made of an invisible energy field, and that thoughts are a creation force that influences this energy field, it's easier to understand how they can play a significant role in the manifestation of the physical things and experiences in your life. Let's explore this science so that you can understand how to use it to create the life of your dreams and cultivate lasting happiness.

First, understand that everything in the universe is made up of energy. All matter (physical objects), including our bodies, are not *really* solid, even though they appear to be. Remember when you were a kid in science class, and you learned how everything in this world is made up of atoms? Maybe you slept through that part of class like I did, but stay with me here, because you're about to see why it's relevant now. Those atoms are made up of tiny particles that are packets of energy. And because everything in the universe is made up of atoms—the trees, your house, your car, your phone—that means everything in this world, even YOU, is made of energy! Your thoughts are also energy. They are a creation force that causes those tiny invisible particles to group together and take physical form.

Let's unpack this further. Your thoughts lead to emotions. And an emotion is really just an energy current in your body, which can also be labeled as a *frequency* or a *vibration*. For example, anger is a frequency, anxiousness is a frequency, sadness is a frequency, and, of course, *happiness is a frequency*. In other words, your thoughts *create* the frequency that you're tuned in to.

> **The frequency you're vibrating at works like a magnet that attracts experiences and objects that match that frequency to eventually appear in your physical reality.**

Your thoughts emit energy into the universal energy field, as well as receive information from the field (we call this inspiration or intuition). This all functions very similar to how a radio works. If you have your radio tuned to a specific station, your radio is receiving the information that is being carried across the ether on *that* frequency. Your brain works the same way. You can be tuned into the frequency of positivity and abundance—where you see the beauty of things, receive inspiration, and make choices in alignment that bring you more positivity and happiness. Or you can be tuned into a frequency of negativity and scarcity—where you see the negative in everything, expect things to go wrong, and make choices that lead to negative outcomes. By now, this is probably starting to add a lot more color as to how the law of attraction works and how you can attract things to you by the frequency you're tapped into, which, again, comes from your thoughts.

This also brings new light to the phrase "vibing with someone." What that really means is you're vibrating on the same frequency as someone, which is why there is an energetic connection that you can feel. This experience is actually a scientific phenomenon labeled spontaneous self-organization. The science behind this is that, when two objects, or people, come together they will often start, after a short period of time, to vibrate together at the same frequency.

I love myself
when I do the little
things that make
me happy.

Sometimes you just cannot vibe with a person no matter how much you might want to. If their frequency is at a lower-level vibration, you will not want to shift to meet them there, but if their frequency is at a higher-level vibration, you will want to be around them, you will want to vibe higher with them. This doesn't make someone a "bad" or "better" person; it is just simply the frequency at which they are vibrating. You can tell how you're vibrating by how you *feel*. So, it's good to stay present and observe how you're feeling at any given moment.

If you aren't sure how to fully be present, let's walk through an exercise together. Wherever you are reading this, take a moment and plant your feet firmly into the ground. Place your palms on your lap facing upward, and (once you've read this) close your eyes, and begin to breathe from the root of your belly all the way up to your chest. Take notice of any tingling in your fingers, soreness in your muscles, or tightness in your chest. Perhaps your eyes feel heavy or you feel a vibration pulsing through your entire body. Whatever comes up for you, breathe into that feeling and into the place it is coming from.

This is an exact practice that you can use to not only shift your energy but also get to know what's going on for you in your body, why it's there, and what it is trying to tell you. This is an amazing practice to do multiple times throughout the day, but you obviously can't do this in the middle of a company meeting or when you're on a conference call. So, here are a few additional mindfulness tools to reference throughout the day.

- Have a mindfulness bell. Have a chime alarm quietly set to go off a few times during the day as a reminder to pause, take a breath, and notice what is around you.

- Create a visual cue for being present. Consider placing a small sticker on your phone, journal, laptop, or refrigerator door to act as a visual reminder to pause and live in the moment. You can also place little notes of affirmations in places around your home that you know you will find throughout the day.

- Take advantage of red lights. Each time you pull up to a red light on the road, use this as a moment to breathe in, notice your feelings and then, if the light is long enough, say something you are grateful for! Be on the lookout throughout your day to take these little pauses that life brings you every day, and use them to your advantage.

- Listen without the intention of responding. If you are in a meeting, worrying about what to say next, or how to respond, it's pretty hard to be fully present. Invite presence into your conversations by listening with curiosity instead of anticipation. This practice of active listening will serve you in not only happiness, but also in speaking your truth. The more you are present, the more you will speak from your heart and from your highest self. When we listen with the intention of pre-scripting ourselves, we open ourselves up to misunderstandings, unspoken truths, and store energy in places that will not be serving us.

The more you practice building in these small moments of presence throughout the day, the easier it will become to turn them into habits that expand not only throughout your entire day, but into all areas of your life. Now that we know more about how to keep ourselves grounded, let's get back to discussing the correlation between our thoughts and our frequency. The frequency you're tuned into creates your physical reality, and your thoughts create the frequency, then you'll probably agree that the thoughts you're thinking are pretty darn important!

Here's the thing, though: 95 percent of our thoughts are subconscious, which means that we are not consciously aware of the majority of the thoughts that go through our mind.

> **We're going through every day operating on these unconscious programs that are constantly running on auto pilot without us even being aware of it.**

And guess what? A lot of these thoughts aren't serving us. They have been conditioned into us from our environment, which includes things such as parents, caregivers, friends, teachers, experiences, messages from childhood, and the media. Let me say it this way: we are NOT consciously creating 95 percent of our thoughts (scary, because we just learned that thoughts create our reality!). Not to worry, though. Fortunately, there are things we can do to impact or influence these subconscious thoughts. And we can condition the right programs that will create the frequencies we'd like to be on.

Probably the most important thing you can do is take conscious control of what you expose your precious mind and attention to throughout your day, every day. In the same way you need to tend to your body daily to take care of it and feed it the right foods to operate at its best, your mind functions in a similar fashion. You need to be careful to make sure it's being exposed to ideas and thoughts that will serve you and empower you rather than take you down. How do you do this? You can read and listen to audiobooks that lift you up. You can also do this by removing negative aspects of your life. You can choose to spend time with people who operate on the frequency you want to be on. If there is a person in your life who always drains you or brings you down, limit the time you spend with them. You can limit your consumption of news and media that focus on spreading fear and negativity.

Another thing you can do is practice gratitude every morning or every night before you go to bed, I love to do both! Write in your journal three things that you are grateful for in your life. Gratitude is the highest frequency you can be on, by the way! Affirmations can be another powerful tool for increasing your frequency. Make a habit of saying positive affirmations to yourself, such as "I am more than enough," or "I deserve love, compassion, and kindness." Don't simply say "I love myself fully and completely," allow yourself to sit still and fully feel yourself fill up with love while you say this affirmation. The key is not just to say the words, but to put emotion behind them when saying them and really *feel* the emotion. Feeling and repetition are the secret sauce when it comes to affirmations.

Now, you may be wondering, "Oh no, if I think a negative thought, does that mean bad things are going to happen to me?" Negative thoughts *will* come up. Don't worry. You're not going to manifest bad things in your reality just by having a couple of thoughts about something. But if you are *living* there, and constantly thinking those thoughts with repetition every day, then you're going to get back the same frequency that you're putting out into the world. Here's what you can do if a negative thought does come up. Simply observe it, honor it, and choose a new positive thought that serves you. We will dive deeper into this in the following chapter (pages 73 to 76).

**See it, believe it, become it.**

I love myself
when I give myself
permission to dream big
and be and do anything
I desire. I am the only
one who needs to believe
in me. Anything more is
just nice to have.

# VISUALIZE YOUR DREAMS
## AND HEAL YOUR PAST THROUGH
## IMAGERY RESCRIPTING

**VISUALIZATION IS A REALLY** powerful tool. It is a form of thought that sends energy and information into the energy field for what you want to experience. Your body can't tell the difference between a real experience and one that is imagined in the mind. Visualization can have real physiological effects on you. With this tool, you can begin to manifest as well as reprogram your experiences and how you responded to them. The reality is that we stimulate the same brain regions when we visualize an action and when we perform that same action. What this means is, when you visualize your goals, your brain doesn't know the difference between actually completing them and visualizing that you are completing them.

Visualization has been a common practice among athletes for years. In fact, one study published in *The American Journal of Clinical Hypnosis* found that nationally ranked Stanford gymnasts were able to complete incredibly complex skills at a much faster rate with improved strength and flexibility simply by incorporating visualization into their training regimen. This isn't only tied to physical feats, entrepreneurs around the world have been known to use visualization to manifest their goals, myself included. I used this exact practice to get over my fear of public speaking. If you are new to this practice and want to start incorporating this tool into your daily life, here are some ways you can begin using visualization as a tool for manifestation.

**STEP 1**

**Be very specific:** To get the most out of your visualization, make it as real as possible. If you want a successful business, visualize the exact colors and design of your office, the financial numbers you meet each quarter and the very specific types of clients you are serving.

**STEP 2**

**Incorporate all your senses:** Visualization isn't only about what you see, but also about including all the senses into your experience. How does the wood of your beautiful work desk feel? What does the scent of your office smell like? What sounds do you hear when you're meeting with a client for the first time?

**STEP 3**

**Be emotional:** Tap into your emotions when you visualize your success. Allow yourself to feel the joy, the love, and happiness that is overflowing your entire being. Fun fact, by adding this emotional experience, you are tapping into your brain's limbic system (the part of the brain involved in our behavioral and emotional responses) making the exercise even more powerful.

**STEP 4**

**Make it a habit:** Frequency is key to getting the most out of visualization. Keep your goals front and center by running through the visualization of your goals at least once a day. I love to practice visualizing my goals each morning to help set my intention for the day. This is a great way to always have your goals in mind! You'll hear me say "set an intention" a lot throughout these chapters, and what I mean by set an intention is, state how you want the day, situation, or whatever it is you are doing to go, what you desire to experience, and who you desire to be. For example, before you step into a meeting, go on a call or walk into a party, set an intention for it:

My intention for this call is for us to resolve.
I will show up powerfully, clear, and direct.

My intention for this party is to have fun,
connect with someone new, and show up fully.

My intention for this day is to experience joy, love,
and to experience abundance.

Now that you have a better idea of how to use visualization for manifesting, let's talk about imagery rescripting for healing. As I mentioned earlier, visualization is a powerful way to manifest your goals and reprogram your experiences. By reprogramming a past experience, you can change the way the experience affected you and affects you currently so you can let go of any pain or trauma that is holding you back from living a joyful life. By doing this technique, you'll understand the power of healing by reprogramming past events through visualization and rescripting. This is an advanced technique used in therapy. I suggest getting support from a therapist or someone trained in this technique to help you dive in, but here is how you can get started using this tool for healing.

To begin to do this, recall an event that was hurtful in the past, one that still has an emotional charge over you. While you imagine the experience from that same age, imagine everything you experienced as detailed and vivid as you possibly can, then step in and begin to rewrite the script. You can imagine something different, maybe it's a different ending, maybe it's something that you needed to hear in that moment that wasn't really said. Be the adult you are and step in to give your inner child what she needed at that moment. Stepping in as your adult self to show up for your inner child is incredibly healing and empowering. You can begin to shift the memory and feelings in your body to rewrite your own story. By rewriting, essentially rescripting your experience, you are creating a different experience for yourself, and changing an experience of pain to one of healing and acceptance. Imagery rescripting is a helpful technique to practice if you are having a hard time moving forward in love because of a hurtful experience from your past.

It is amazing what science can do and how the science of happiness can work to heal parts of you, reprogram, and improve your inner and outer world. You are worth this work, you are worthy of rewriting any parts of your story that do not serve you. Be the person who you needed, that is loving yourself. Give yourself what you needed at that moment of that experience so that you can move forward in healing and let go of any negative feelings,

> **When you rise, everyone around you will rise, and you will make the impact in the world you are meant to create.**

# 15 WAYS TO CULTIVATE HAPPINESS

**1** **Confront your negative feelings.** When you confront your negative feelings head on, you are confronting your fears and letting go of what is not serving you.

**2** **Do things that make you happy.** To create lasting happiness, you have to practice doing things that create little pockets of happiness, like shopping or going skiing, or going to the beach.

**3** **Cultivate your purpose.** When you find what you are passionate about, pursue that. Part of being happy is living a life full of purpose and part of doing that is doing things that bring out the spark inside of you. Only you know what creates meaning for you in your life and what sparks your passion.

**4** **Know your values.** Part of loving yourself is knowing who you are at the core. As I've said before, your values are constantly evolving as you are and it's important to check in with them and know what they are. When you know what your values are, you are clear on what you want.

**5** **Spend time doing the things you value.** If you value your family, spend more time with them. If you value expression, do the thing that allows you to express yourself freely. When you honor something that has deep meaning for you, you are giving yourself the space to know more about yourself and what is important to you.

**6** **Practice shifting negative thoughts into positive thinking.** Thoughts have a powerful way of creating our realities and when we stay in a negative funk, we are not allowing opportunities and positive things to enter our lives.

**7** **Build more small moments of presence.** The more you practice grounding yourself by taking time to breathe or creating a visual cue for being present, the easier it will be to turn these into habits.

**8** **Actively listen.** Listening with the intention of responding will just create a mountain of anxiety about what you are going to say or create tons of swirling thoughts about how you will respond instead of giving yourself the chance to respond from your truest self. When you practice actively listening, not only are you respecting the other person, but also you are giving yourself the chance to speak from the heart, so you can have a more meaningful conversation.

**9** **Say positive affirmations to yourself with feeling and repetition.** Believe and feel what you are saying about yourself so that you can cultivate a loving relationship with yourself. When you believe in yourself, you are unstoppable.

**10** **Take conscious control of what you expose your mind and body to.** Feed your body nutritious foods and expose your mind to empowering thoughts and ideas. Practice being thankful, listen to uplifting audio books, and say positive affirmations to yourself.

**11** **Visualize your dreams.** By visualizing your desires, you are putting them out into the universe and one step closer to creating the reality you envision.

**12** **Make visualizing your goals a habit.** If you do this for yourself often, you will always be able to manifest what you want out of life. At the very least, you will always cultivate confidence and allow yourself to receive the gifts of the universe.

**13** **Create meaningful intentions for yourself.** To manifest what you want, first you have to be clear about what it is that you want and be as specific as possible about your desires.

**14** **Rescript past memories.** Again, I do recommend doing this with the help of a professional, but there are ways for you to start doing this. Be the person that you needed at the moment and recreate your memory for healing.

**15** **Show up for yourself.** Be the person that you wished someone was for you when you were younger. Be the person that you are to your loved one when they need you. When you show up for yourself, you are showing yourself ultimate kindness and love.

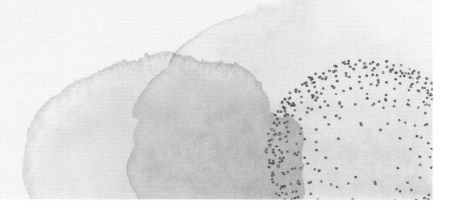

## Homework: Value Your Worth

### YOUR INVITATION

*I invite you to simply be available to see yourself reflected through the science of happiness and taking care of yourself. If you can, you are going to get so much out of it by being able to deepen your understanding of who you are, what you need, and how you can best meet those needs. It can prescriptively construct your self-care and deepen your inner love. We don't always need to know how things work—that is sometimes the joy of this journey and expanding our minds.*

Part of valuing your worth means making things that are important to you a priority. Let's dive further into your values and also how you can create a higher frequency into your life as well as bring in more joy so that you can be living on a high frequency and manifesting the things you desire into your life from that frequency.

**Step 1:** Take some time to think about things that are important to you. What are five things that are most important to you in life? Rank them as best you can on level of importance. Next to each, write down what feeling it creates for you. For example, if the feeling is joy, then having fun could be a value of yours.

**Step 2:** What are just three things that you stand for? For example, I stand for equal rights, honesty, and freedom, to name a few. Next to each of the three things on your list, write down what characteristics are needed. For example, if you put honesty, then some characteristics could be truthfulness and integrity. Therefore, truthfulness and integrity are part of your values and you will want to lead with those qualities in your life and surround yourself with people who also have those qualities.

**Step 3:** After you've taken some time to explore what your values are, create a gratitude board. Vision boards are all the rage, but part of manifesting your vision and goals is being grateful for what you already have. Creating a gratitude board supports you in vibing at the frequency of love so that you can quickly manifest more of it into your life. Another thing that a gratitude board will do for you is remind you how far you've come and what you have already manifested, and it will instill belief and

possibility in you. When you are focused on what you don't yet have or focused on the next goal, you can lose sight of how much you have accomplished. This puts you into goal mode without praising and acknowledging what you have already created. You miss out on the experience of being proud of yourself and showing yourself that you really can do anything. So, create a board of all the things that you are proud of and grateful for in your life and reflect on how you got here. This is an instant hack for confidence and high frequency.

**Higher Love Level:** For some extra high vibes into your days, get a small circle of friends or your family (kids love this practice) and celebrate your wins from the week. Each person can take 2 minutes and share what they are grateful from their week, and after each person's turn, cheer for them like they just won the Superbowl or an Oscar. This creates a high frequency around you and them, as well as getting you and anyone involved more excited about life and more motivated to create wins in their days.

> **Be open to the path that is waiting to take you higher, daily.**

# I ONLY SPEAK LOVE OVER MYSELF

# Chapter 3

# THE FOUR PROMISES

**OUR TRUE NATURE** is love, but somewhere along the way, usually in childhood, outside events cause us to leave this state of living behind. We find ourselves feeling inadequate, lonely, and filled with fear.

I had a client. Let's call her Mary. When she was a little girl, she was an incredibly gifted piano player. One day, she sat down at a piano, stared at the black and white keys, and voilà! She simply knew how to play. She would rush home every day after school, eager to write new songs, filling the house with her music. One afternoon, she sat down to compose a new song. She played the same few measures over and over, working to get the notes out exactly as she heard them in her head. Her mother stormed into the living room and boomed, "Knock it off, I can't work with all of this obnoxious noise!" Mary's fingers shook over the keys. Her shoulders hunched over the piano and doubt filled her mind. Her music wasn't welcome. It wasn't valued. So, she stopped.

What she learned later was that her mother loved hearing her play. It was just that on that day she was overworked and had let stress get the better of her. Her mother had no idea the impact her actions would have. Unfortunately, this brief moment in time changed Mary. She not only stopped playing music, but she also began to hide her talents, to quiet her inner strength, and to step away from her carefree natural state of being. She didn't realize what she was doing—she just thought she was keeping everyone around her at peace.

You may be carrying a story like this deep within you. You may have a hidden memory of being a joyful, bold, and confident child, who, by a mistake, a misstep, or a misunderstanding, is replaced with someone afraid, ashamed, and confused about how to step out into the world.

And here's the thing—once we start down this path, we keep going, repeating those same mistakes without even realizing it. That little girl didn't just stop playing piano: she stopped making any noise at all, she never played the piano again and instead became a writer. She often thinks about music and writes beautiful words, but she doesn't dare try to play them. We do the same, throughout our lives. We get thrown out of our natural state of love, and then we keep throwing ourselves out, over and over again. We quiet ourselves.

But it is possible to step off that path and return to that beautiful state of love. It requires breaking down these old patterns and rediscovering a new set of ideals, celebrating our own joyful songs.

I have found that there are four promises you can make to yourself, four standards to live by, so that you can spend every day in love with you. We'll come back to these promises again and again throughout this book. Finding your way back to love isn't easy, but it is possible, and these promises can serve as lodestones, as four lanterns to light your way. They are a code, a way to create a life you love.

Your willingness to open this book and begin this journey is the beginning of setting these standards. Before we dive into each promise, take out a notebook and pen and write: *I am ready to love myself. These four promises are my pathway to loving me.* Then write the following four promises to yourself.

I am unavailable for comparison.

I am unavailable to be mean to me any longer.

I am committed to myself and to my dreams, first.

I trust myself.

# I AM UNAVAILABLE FOR COMPARISON

**MY FINGERS ARE** trembling as I begin this story, because I know how much it changed me, and how much a story like this likely changed you.

I was in first grade and a friend from class was having a slumber party for her birthday. My parents weren't quite sure I was old enough for a slumber party, but I desperately wanted to go, so I boldly outlined a list of reasons why I should be allowed to. As usual, this boldness in me was met with displeasure, but they reluctantly agreed to let me go to the party.

The moment their heads nodded yes, I ran into my cozy bedroom and packed my little pink suitcase with plastic wheels full of dress-up clothes even though the sleepover wasn't for another three days. I was so excited I could barely sleep on the nights leading up to it. The day finally came, and my parents drove me up the long driveway to my friend's house.

I stood outside her home, stunned. It was giant. I thought it looked like a Disney castle. I walked into the party and it was just a blur of fancy foods, a backyard the size of our school playground, and bedrooms that felt larger than my whole house. And it wasn't just the house that was fancy; *they* were fancy. They had giant portraits of themselves on the walls of their hallway, and they were all dressed so well and looked so good.

More than anything, I felt how easily they fit together. They all seemed so happy and loving. Watching my friend open her birthday presents with all her relatives circled around, I wondered, "Why wasn't my family like this? Why wasn't I good enough to have all of this?"

I had always remembered my parents doing everything they could do to make our birthdays special, even when they couldn't afford it, but with each hug they gave each other, I shrank into myself. I was naturally confident, but when I compared myself with everything they had, I felt so small. When I went home the next morning, the bedroom that I loved felt like a shoebox, and the love I looked for between my parents didn't match what I had seen at my friend's house.

This was just a fleeting moment, and soon enough I stepped back into myself . . . and yet, this act of comparison became part of my nature. From that moment on, I constantly checked myself against others, whether it was my looks, my intelligence, my talent, my possessions—everything I was and everything I had was measured against other people.

I know I am not alone in this. We all do it, consciously or unconsciously. It's part of what it is to be a woman, as we are told who we "should" and "shouldn't" be. I was told I was "too much" so often that it became a reference point in my brain. I formed the unconscious belief that my natural state of being wasn't "right" or good enough—and the conclusion I came to was that I had better look to see how other people were so I could copy them, so I could be good enough.

Once you start course-correcting yourself based on what other people are doing, you create a habit of looking outside of yourself for who you should be. I have seen this in every corner of life. Kids model after one another, mothers compare their mothering skills with other moms, men compare their skill sets with other men—and suddenly here we are, forming a society that is constantly living in a state of comparison. Everyone has abandoned their natural gifts and unique perspectives in order to fit what is "normal" and "right."

Social media has only made all of this that much worse. Before we would compare ourselves with others when we saw them in person, but now we can scroll through the lives of people all over the world, including people with some pretty unrelatable experiences. Instead of a friend with a large home that seems like a castle, you've got dozens of actual castles available for comparison at a moment's notice. You are watching what strangers are doing with their day, in their relationships, in their careers.

Worst of all, it's not *really* what they're doing. It's what they are choosing to show you, and like everyone, they want to show off only the very best parts of themselves—or more accurately, what they in their own swamp of comparison *believe* is the best and most successful.

**Never forget that social media is nothing more than a snapshot into someone's life. You are viewing one perfect moment captured in the midst of an imperfect day.**

There is a story and journey behind it all. But we take these images for truth and believe that's what a perfect life should look like. It's not real life, but we still set it as an unattainable goal, and punish ourselves when we don't meet it. Sure, sometimes we have our own Instagram-worthy moments that look like the perfect life, but those moments are fleeting and exhausting, and honestly? They probably aren't even real. They don't bring true joy.

All this comparison leaves you unfulfilled, unhappy, and unsatisfied. It can make you feel miserable about your life and exhausted by constantly trying to live up to an image or ideal that likely isn't even real. It feels as though all that someone else has accomplished is yet another shiny billboard flashing in your eyes as you drive home telling yourself that you aren't good enough, that you can't make your dreams come true. Comparison only breeds more comparison, creating more separation and disconnection from ourselves and our natural state of love.

I struggled so hard with this for so much of my life. It's not really a surprise. Most people who have a brand or a company that has anything to do with helping people focus their teachings around their own experiences, or what they would have wanted to know back when they were stuck in the mess. I had been this little girl whose natural state was sassy independence, but who somehow, along the way, made so many people uncomfortable, just by being authentically herself. My natural way of living life became a story of other people's discomfort, and that was the door that allowed comparison to creep in. People are often uncomfortable with what they don't understand or can't quite label, but what I know now is that this discomfort is their problem, not mine—and it isn't yours either!

I spent so much of my life in a state of comparison, looking outside myself to know how to live, and it was exhausting. Living on the other side, bravely and unapologetically as my authentic self, has given me so much freedom, pleasure, and love. All I want is for you to live this way too. The good news is you can break free from this destructive cycle.

**It will take some time, but by making small choices every day to grow and retrain your brain, teaching it to view life through a different lens, one that focuses less on the negative and more on gratitude in your life, you will move forward step by step into your own beautiful bravery.**

I love myself
when I stop comparing
myself to others.

This starts with awareness. We don't even realize how much time we spend comparing ourselves to others, and if you put some attention on it, you will quickly understand just how much energy, time, and joy comparison has been sucking out of your life. But tread lightly, as the last thing you need is to start judging yourself for participating in a culture that has surrounded you from childhood. *Of course* you've been comparing. It's what you were taught to do. Unlearning that way of life will take some time, and to be honest, the urge to compare will always be there, but you can choose to ignore it and move past it.

**As you begin to notice yourself starting to compare to others, promise yourself that you will do it from a place of love and compassion.**

The root of your comparison is likely that you want to live a bold and fulfilling life, which is so amazing! Up to now, the only way you've known how to reach for that life is by comparing yourself to others . . . but now you can reach for more.

For one week, pay attention to your comparison habits. What are you comparing? Is it social media pages with large followings? Is it your health and physical appearance? Is it your relationship status? Is it your wealth or abundance? Write them down in your journal. This may be uncomfortable, but this is valuable information! Do your best to view your comparison with curiosity instead of judgment, as you learn more about the desires behind your comparisonitis.

For the month following this week, practice adjusting your attitude. Instead of thinking from a place of lack with thoughts like "Why don't I have that?" refocus your thoughts to more positive thinking like "I am available and receiving all the gifts the universe has in store for me."

If you've been having trouble with social media, pay attention to that. We often check our social media feeds mindlessly, while standing in line at a coffee shop or sitting in traffic. Try something: before signing on, set an intention for positivity. Tell yourself, "I'm going to find inspiration here," and then when you see those fitness models working out or those gorgeous travel pictures, view it as a source of inspiration to guide you on your path, not derail you from it.

Or if the source of your comparisonitis is a friend that you feel envious of, take some time to unpack that. Where is this coming from? Is it something she is doing, intentionally or otherwise? If so, maybe take a break from each other. But if it comes entirely from you, look closely at what it is you're envying. What does this say about what you want in life? How can you step away from comparison and move instead to pursuing your dreams?

The overstimulation of social media and being blasted with what everyone else is doing can make our comparison compass go crazy, its needle spinning all around, until we no longer have any idea of what we truly want. You can't avoid comparing yourself with others. We can work on unlearning this behavior, but it's so deeply ingrained that you are going to come back to it from time to time. When that happens, just be aware of it. Remember that it's natural, and then take a step back from it.

The practice of unlearning comparison is similar to the practice of meditating. When you're meditating, you're not actually supposed to *not think*. Every time you try, you end up thinking about not thinking. Instead, let any thoughts that come up make their way across your mind, and then let them go. The same strategy can work when you're caught up in comparing yourself to others. "Okay," you say to yourself, "I'm comparing now." And then let the thought go. Redirect yourself to *you*. When you're having negative thoughts about yourself and what you like, bring yourself back to you by thinking something positive about yourself. Focus on abundance, rather than on lack. Instead of saying, "I am not enough because I don't have what they have," think, "I am enough. I am running my own race, and I will get there." You will get there the way you are meant to because you are not her, you are *you*. Your path is sacred to you and you only, there is always enough for all of us and the way you get there will be different from anyone else, trust and embrace which way is meant for you.

Right now, commit to this: *I'm unavailable for comparison.* Say it over and over again if you need to, because the last person that is going to stand in your way is yourself.

# The Four A's to Get Out of Comparisonitis

It is not easy to not compare. But what does all this comparison do? It can make you feel miserable about your life and leave you exhausted from constantly trying to live up to an image or idea that likely isn't even real. One of the things that continued to come up in my speaking events and in my workshops was comparison, especially with social media! I recently traveled to different cities to speak on various news channels about how to get out of comparison. Use what I call the four A's to prevent yourself from going into comparisonitis:

**Awareness:** Catch comparison before it turns into a loop. To simply be aware and catch yourself in comparison is a tool to stop and examine where it comes from.

**Acceptance:** Accept that those thoughts come up and comparison has been ingrained in us. This is something we must unlearn, and the more we are focused on filling ourselves up the less intense comparison will be.

**Affirmations:** When you catch yourself in comparison, affirmations and self-talk can support you. For example, you could say to yourself: "That is perfect for them, this has nothing to do with me. I am beautiful, special, and on my own path."

**Action:** Many times, we spot things we want, go into comparison, and stay there, creating a negative thought loop that leads to a domino effect of self-doubt. When you are in comparison, ask yourself the necessary questions and then take the action needed to get out of the comparison trap.

Ask yourself:

Why is this bothering me?

Do I want this? Why?

Is this true?

What can I do to make myself feel better about this?

How does this have nothing to do with me?

The only thing comparison does is kill your dreams and your focus. It takes you off your path. Refocus and get back to leading the life you're dreaming of.

I love myself when I focus on leading the life of my dreams.

# I AM UNAVAILABLE
# TO BE MEAN TO ME ANY LONGER

**WHEN I WAS** growing up, I wanted my family to love me for who I was, but at the same time, I couldn't help but wonder if who I was, was "right." Every day felt like a struggle to be the person they wanted me to be, and back then I felt as if I failed at it. My thoughts were a constant repeat of "You aren't doing it right" and "They want you to be this way . . . why can't you just do it?" Every time I spoke or did anything, whether it was voicing my opinion or helping someone in need, I would hesitate. "Is this what they want me to do?" I walked around wondering why I couldn't be who they wanted me to be.

Being hard on ourselves is a pattern we rely on. We are told to be a certain way, and when we fail, we abuse ourselves with negative self-talk in order to get ourselves to do better next time. Beneath your negative self-talk is a wound that may have been caused by even the most minor or insignificant moment, sparking the negative pattern. Someone made fun of your outfit in middle school, so you forever question your fashion sense and hate how you look leaving the house each day. Your first partner cheated on you, and since then, you have only dated men who are distant, avoidant, and distracted. You always wanted to be a singer and didn't get into the high school musical, and now you protect yourself from pursuing other dreams because they seem silly and almost absurd. I always wanted to be an activist and a performer, and the constant reminder to lower my light held me back for years.

Negative self-talk can look like a lot of things. It can sound subtle ("I'm not great at doing math, so I shouldn't volunteer for this work project . . . don't want to embarrass myself!"). Or it can be downright mean ("There is no use, I'll never be good enough."). These thoughts might seem minor, but they create some pretty painful outcomes in your life. The reality is, rumination and self-blame over painful events have been found to be linked to an increased risk of mental health problems. It's true. Our thoughts can literally make us sick. But the good news is that the reverse is also true.

A Japanese doctor, Masaru Emoto, was able to demonstrate the power of human thought by experimenting with water. He exposed one glass of water to emotions and sounds of gratitude and love, and separately exposed a different glass of water, from the same source, to negative thoughts, with heavy metal music and sadness. As the water froze, he took pictures that captured the crystals of the water as they formed. The water exposed to positive and uplifting words and music formed beautiful symmetrical snowflake crystals, while the water exposed to the angry and sad sounds formed jagged and scattered shapes.

**When you consider that almost 60 percent of our bodies are composed of water, that means the thoughts we direct at ourselves play a huge role in changing us on a cellular level.**

Negative thoughts have been a part of your life for a long time, so they won't just disappear the moment you decide they aren't welcome anymore. But the moment they show up, you can cut them off immediately, replacing them with a new and improved perspective. You can begin to head them off at the pass by writing positive phrases on sticky notes or repeating positive phrases to yourself—anything positive that you can do can reverse the cycle. For instance, if you find yourself thinking things like, "Ugh, I look a mess again today," write out a note that says, "Hello, gorgeous!" You can keep these on your bathroom mirror, on the back of your phone, on your refrigerator—wherever you will see them and notice them. And then, whenever you see them, say them *out loud.* Sure, it'll feel silly at first, but verbalizing and allowing yourself to hear these phrases will make them louder, helping them drown out the negative thoughts.

A study published on ScienceDirect showed that athletes who uttered motivational affirmations to themselves while they played performed better than those who stayed silent. Well, guess what? It's game time, ladies! For an extra boost, consider using your full name with your affirmation. So instead of saying, "I am healthy, strong, and beautiful," I say, "Sarah is healthy, strong, and beautiful." Again, this feels super awkward at first, but using your name out loud has been proven to help reframe negative self-talk by providing a more objective view. Giving yourself a little space helps you take a more compassionate approach. We're working on getting you to be your own best friend. All you're doing here is saying "hi!".

Life is filled with so many things we can't control—unforeseeable events, unplanned emergencies, and the circumstances we are born into. But there are some things we *can* control, such as our thoughts. Now, we can *know* this on an intellectual level, but actually releasing negative self-talk can be a little more difficult. In many ways, it can feel like saying goodbye to a friend you have become so comfortable with, but that you know, deep down, is not good for you. Your heart and gut are telling you to move on, but releasing this part of yourself feels like a loss. Being mean to yourself sometimes feels sort of *good*, doesn't it? Negative self-talk has been there for you when you've been trying to do better, trying to work harder, trying to make other people happy—all things that we genuinely want, that are good things to want! The problem is that while negative self-talk is intended to help us get those things, it doesn't. In reality, it just makes it harder for us to be happy and successful at being *us*.

> **Inner confidence comes from choosing to be brave enough to believe you are worthy of it all.**

No matter how many battles I fought with my father, and no matter how many times I chastised myself for not being able to be less than all that I am, I could never put out the fire that burned within my soul. My spirit just wouldn't die, despite my attempts to kill it, and for that I am forever grateful. Underneath it all, you are that beautifully brave version of yourself, and no matter how much you try to push her down, she is still there, aching to be set free.

**Release the negative self-talk. Release you.**

Begin to consciously acknowledge the negative thoughts and voices that creep into your mind. It will be so tempting to let them sneak in, but choose to confront them. Turn them away at the door like the unwelcome visitors they are. A process that I take my clients and any of my event attendees through (and use myself) is a process I call "flip it." It's a practice of flipping a negative thought into a positive one. Try this technique the next time you notice a repeated negative thought or worry loop come up. Write down the thought or worry in your journal and then next to it write an opposite thought. Sometimes, you might find yourself doing up to five thoughts at a time.

Notice it. Honor it. Get curious about it. Say to yourself, "[Your Name], I love you, I am so sorry this keeps coming up. This is from [linked past event]. I am curious as to why it's still here, what is it showing me?" Then choose and declare a new thought. What is your new thought?

| If you often tell yourself: | Try this narrative: |
|---|---|
| "I'm not good enough for that . . ." | "I am more than enough as I am. I am doing something new that takes time to master." |
| "I don't have the resources to do this." | "I will always find a way." |
| "It's going to be one of those days . . ." | "Everything works out in my favor. I am stepping into the happiest and most amazing days of my life." |
| "There is no point: I'll lose weight and then gain it right back again." | "The past does not define me. I am healthy, strong, and beautiful." |

I love myself
when I choose to be
brave enough to believe
I am worth it all.

# I AM COMMITTED TO MYSELF
# AND TO MY DREAMS, FIRST

**BURNOUT SUCKS.** We are conditioned from a young age to be everything to everyone. We must be a supportive friend, a hardworking employee, a nurturing mother, a loving wife, a dutiful daughter . . . the list goes on and on. And when we toss in our own personal goals of building a brand, starting a passion hustle, or creating art, there is just *so much.* Maybe too much.

And what do we do? We say yes to everything! We are women, we can do it all! In reality, we shouldn't. Yes, you are one strong queen, but when you try to literally do it all, you are doomed to failure. The things you want most do not get the full attention they need, and everything starts to feel half-hearted. You start to feel overwhelmed and maybe even resentful that you don't have the time to work on the thing you really love, even personal relationships can start to suffer. And when you try, you're not able to show up as your best self. If you try to please everyone, you'll end up pleasing no one.

A while ago, I was grabbing a matcha latte from one of my favorite cafes when I bumped into a friend. I asked how she was doing, and her response was, "Things are great! I'm not too busy and have found such a balance with free time and doing work." I froze and my head tilted back. *Say what?* I couldn't remember the last time I had heard the words *great* and *not busy* in the same sentence. The women in my life tend to complain (well, humble-brag) about how busy they are and how little free time they have for anything leisure, as if that is some sort of symbol of their worth. We have begun to equate our worth with how much free time we *don't* have. Sounds kind of backward when you think about it like that, doesn't it?

I asked my friend how on earth she was managing such a thing. How was she able to be successful (and I knew she was) *and* have free time? She told me something that blew my mind. She said she'd started to fall in love with the word *no.* It's such a powerful word, and it's not one that we're used to. It feels rude. There's an old part of me that sometimes clenches up at the thought of it. It feels like it goes against everything we are taught about how we ought to be in the world. But it is necessary—and not only that, it's the *right thing to do, for you.*

> **Saying NO is just as important as saying YES.**

It takes practice, and it will get easier with time. At the beginning, though, it can be hard to sort through. If you never say "no," how do you know where to begin? Start by taking a really close look at the things you are saying "yes" to. If your calendar is anything like mine, it's color-coded with all the things you "have" to do each week. The first thing I began to change was my relationship with the phrase *have to*. Looking at your calendar, what are those things, and more importantly, *why* do you do them? Understanding why you take the actions you take can be the fastest way to eliminating commitments that don't align with your life. If you are saying "yes" to things because you feel guilty, or because something feels like an obligation, or you know you will be judged if you don't, then that is definitely something you can start saying "no" to. And then, once you've cleared up some space, what can you choose to say "yes" to? This takes just as much discernment and thought as saying "no." Every "yes" you give is a commitment to yourself, and so is every "no." What's that saying again? "No" is a complete sentence. I like to say that not only is "no" a complete sentence, but it's also a bouncer for your burnout.

So how to choose?

> Here's what I have come to believe about living fully in love with yourself: you must focus on one big goal at a time.

I know, this is so hard to accept, especially if, like me, you are a dreamer who's always thinking things like, "I want to be an author, a coach, a podcast host, and start a family all in one year!"

I promise, there is absolutely a way to have everything in the end. But to get there, you have to choose which of your dreams and goals matter the most to you, which one to focus on first. Which one will have the largest impact on your life this year? Make that choice, and then focus on that singular goal with all of your power and soul.

Otherwise, you are 100 percent going to hit burnout. Even if everything you are doing is *for you*, even if you are passionate and working on your dreams, if you don't take control of your time and manage it, you are going to get overwhelmed. You are an amazing, powerful, vibrant woman, but there's just one of you, and there are only so many hours in the day. Some of those hours need to be spent sleeping. Others need to be spent having fun and relaxing! Your time is *yours*. Make sure you are using it wisely and with love for yourself. Getting to this point takes practice and careful consideration. The following four steps will help you reduce unnecessary calendar clutter, reprioritize your time, and find true value in every single day.

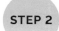

### Track your calendar for a week.

**STEP 1**

It's time to get very detailed with your calendar! From the moment you wake up to the moment you go to sleep at night, track your day in 15-minute intervals. Do your best to pick a week that is very "standard" to your usual living setup. If you are going on a vacation or have an unusual work event during the week, then perhaps wait. If a scattered schedule is normal, track a few weeks at this pace to get a better idea of how things look.

This may sound intense, but trust me, you will quickly realize how you are spending your time, and you'll find lots of information about whether it's how you *want* to be spending your time. Color-code your calendar as you track it so you can understand it at a glance. (Here's how I do it—work: yellow; fitness: blue; meals: purple, etc.).

### Review and adjust.

**STEP 2**

After a week of tracking your calendar meticulously, dedicate an evening to review everything. Get comfy and treat this as positive you-time. Make it a self-care celebration! Review where the majority of your time has gone and get as granular as possible. If you have "work" all day (which most of us do), then identify which projects, actions, or tasks you are doing most often. Do the same with your leisure time, time spent with friends, and time spent with family—again, get granular. Then list them out in order of most time to least time. Next to each item, write why you do it and how it makes you feel.

For a lot of us, that will include a lot of things we don't like doing that make us feel pretty bad. And that's great! Wait, what? Yes. This is good news because it means you've found tasks that you should absolutely cut down on or get rid of entirely. Say you discovered you spend twelve hours a week on social media, or six hours a week in meetings for a project that isn't going anywhere. Perhaps you realized that you spend seven hours attending happy hours with friends whom you don't actually like all that much.

These are golden nuggets to help you get back on track and remove what isn't serving you.

### What *do* you want?

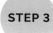

Okay, so you've figured out what you're doing that you don't want to be doing any longer. Now ask yourself: "What *do* I want?" Now is the time to prioritize. Spend another evening—this one will be *much* more fun, I promise!—writing out a list of your goals and dreams. Enjoy this and get as detailed as you can.

When you're done, rank them! What's most important to you? What do you want to focus on first? There will be a lot of factors to consider, including timeline, financial options, outside responsibilities, and so forth, so take your time. Each and every one of them is possible, so it's just a matter of figuring out what you want to put your attention on first.

This is about *you* and what *you want.* Show your love for yourself by choosing things that will best serve you.

### Commit and say no.

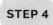

With a clear understanding of where your time is spent in relation to the goals you have for yourself, it's time to commit to change. Look at saying "no" as though it is a gift to yourself. Each "no" is a gift of a "yes" to something that will serve you. Start small if you need to and begin to remove one item from your life that isn't serving you—just one. If you spent your entire Tuesday evening with friends who didn't lift you up, having margaritas that left you feeling bad, consider forgoing this commitment altogether, or only attend on special occasions. There! You just gifted yourself an entire night to do something you truly love!

This won't always be easy. I get it. People have come to have certain expectations of you, and all of a sudden, you're saying "no"? But here's the thing: you were very careful about what you chose to say "no" to. You chose things that weren't good for you. And if these people love you as you love yourself, they will completely get that. If not? Well, then that just makes the decision that much easier.

I love myself when I refuse to sell myself short for anyone else's approval. I see my value, know my worth, and declare my evolution.

# I TRUST MYSELF

**YOU ARE FAR MORE** powerful and intelligent than you think. This isn't me being your cheerleader—although I totally am!—this is based on science. Consider this: Have you ever gotten that feeling when you walk into a room, and something just feels . . . off? A shiver runs down your spine and you feel a flutter in your core, but you aren't sure why. Nothing is glaringly wrong, so you push it down and stay where you are.

While your conscious brain is busy talking to people, ordering a drink, or responding to a text message, your intuitive right brain is "reading" your surroundings and sending you subtle messages. It spotted something you didn't consciously notice, and it turns out the creepy guy from the office next door is there at the bar.

This is also sometimes referred to as your gut instinct. When someone asks, "What does your gut tell you?" there's a reason for that! The gut is often called "the second brain." It contains more than two million nerves, more than your actual brain has. The nerves in your gut act as a truth teller, guiding you toward what is a "yes" and what is a "no" in your life. This second brain communicates directly to your primary brain through a network of neurons, chemicals, and hormones, and this superhighway allows the brain and the gut to be constantly updating one another. This is why there is such a drastic connection between gastrointestinal issues and mental health. Studies have begun to show that conditions such as irritable bowel syndrome (IBS), constipation, bloating, and upset stomach may be the cause of anxiety and depression, not necessarily the other way around. When your intuitive second brain is upset, it may be sending signals to the central nervous system that changes your mood. So truly, your gut is telling your mind what is right and wrong on both a physiological and an intuitive level.

Have you ever noticed that women in particular really seem to be connected to their intuition? We just know when things are off in a relationship, or when it feels like something troubling is on the horizon. This beautiful gift is not your imagination. It is rooted in science, as women have been found to have a higher capacity for connecting to their intuitive senses on a physiological level. Women's connective white matter (corpus colosseum), the part of the brain that connects our left and right brain hemispheres, is thicker compared to that of men. This highway of the brain is at hyper speed for women, allowing us to access our intuition faster and more powerfully. But it only works if we're listening. In order to catch these trusty signals, you must be present in the moment, paying attention. What are your instincts saying? If you're aware, they speak to you loud and clear.

I have found that gauging whether something is right for me is actually surprisingly simple. When I first met Josh, I knew in my soul that he was my husband. Does that sound crazy romantic? Maybe, but it's the truth. I just *felt* it, and it was as simple as that. This feeling was like instant calm. It's like certainty and connection and a whisper from the soul. *This is your person.*

Does that mean I listened to my intuition right away? Yeah, not really. Like most people, I ignored my gut and went in the opposite direction. We were so clearly right for each other that friends and family could see it too, but I gave every excuse I could think of, claiming he wasn't the one for me. Why? Because of fear. Because the thought, "What if it doesn't work out?" had begun to creep in. We are paralyzed by fear. Fear is our single greatest oppressor. It is the thing that stands in the way of everything we want in life.

We are afraid of love, because what if it doesn't last? We are afraid of success, because what if we fail? We are afraid of happiness, because what if, when it's gone, we are devastated?

Our biggest fear, the sum of all of these, is to be fully alive. I have found that the closest feeling to joy is fear. They are two sides of the same coin. We can be so frightened by our own potential, by the risk of fully living and expressing who we really are, that we stop ourselves from doing what we know deep down is right because we are in fear of losing it if we do. A lot of that fear comes down to our limiting beliefs. We've picked up these beliefs, often in childhood, and they aren't ours and they aren't real, but we carry them around with us anyway. Beliefs like "I'm not enough," "This kind of thing doesn't happen for people like me," and "It's not going to last." These beliefs and the fear behind them are always there, controlling us. They keep us from taking risks, whether that's starting a new relationship, putting yourself forward for a promotion, or starting that business you've always dreamed of.

I used to always think five steps ahead, like I was living in an eternal chess match. "If I do this, then this will happen, which means this will happen, and then that can happen, and finally this will happen." If I couldn't see all the way to the end of those five steps, then I couldn't be sure things would work out, and so I wouldn't even try.

Now, you know as well as I do that hardly anything worth doing can possibly be that planned out. And even if you *make* those plans, odds are something you didn't anticipate will happen. That's for sure how it happened for me most of the time! But I couldn't stop myself—my fear was controlling me, and it kept me from moving forward.

Here's the thing, though: you never hear someone at the end of their life say, "Whew, I'm sure glad I didn't go after that dream/tell that guy how I felt/go on that adventure!" The regrets we have are the risks we *didn't* take, the experiences we didn't have.

**When we cut ourselves off from possibility, we are cutting ourselves off from experiencing life at its fullest. On the other side of fear is what your soul is meant to experience.**

When I tell you to be brave, I'm not saying don't be afraid. I'm not saying you can wave some magic wand and sparkle away those limiting beliefs. Fear is always going to show up in your life. Bravery means living with fear.

You have the choice to walk through that fear. It takes 90 seconds for a feeling to progress through your body, but most of the time, we don't even give ourselves that much time. We experience fear and we clamp down on it hard, clutching it in tight. A study published by *Psychology Today* explains how brain scientist Jill Bolte Taylor studies and reports on our ability to regulate the neurological process that she calls "the 90-second rule." I study this "90-second rule," working with it in myself and empowering my clients to use it and get curious about it. Let's break this rule down; when you experience an emotion, say sadness, your body has a physiological reaction for at most 90 seconds. After this sensation passes, any time spent remaining in that emotion is your choice. You are choosing to stay in that emotion. So, what if you decided to let yourself *feel* that fear? What if you let it have its moment, and then you took the first step to walk through it? I am so grateful that my intuition overcame my fear. It wasn't easy; in the beginning, I did just about everything I could to sabotage my relationship with Josh! I was so scared. But there was a force stronger than me that kept us together despite everything. In the end, my intuition was so insistent that I took the risk, and I thank her every day. Josh is my best friend and my biggest healer.

All of those voices in your mind, all those limiting beliefs, will drown out your intuition—and it will be easy, because negativity screams at you, while intuition comes like a quiet whisper, one you have to really pay attention to. But know this—it always speaks first. Your intuition is always the first thing that comes up . . . but then you go on to drown it out with doubt and fear. If you're feeling stuck, go back to the beginning. That's where the real answers are.

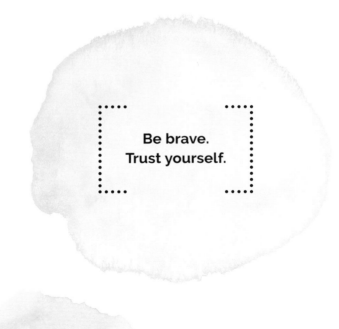

Be brave.
Trust yourself.

After spending years learning how to silence and tone down your intuition, it can be hard to reconnect. Intuition communicates in different ways for different people, but it is often connected to a primary sense. For me, it feels physical, like a knot in my stomach or goosebumps blooming over my skin. You might receive visual stimulation, like a blurring at the edges of your vision or even a slowing down of time, like you're watching your life in slow motion. You might hear a ringing in your ears or an echoing sound. However it comes, if you've ever felt you knew the truth in the depths of your soul, it is a message from your intuition.

Your intuition may even show up at certain times during the day. When you're facing a difficult choice and you wake up after "sleeping on it," you may feel a sense of clarity. Others feel more grounded and connected in the middle of the night, as they are either awakened at 2 a.m. with what they know to be true or as they receive messages in their dreams. We are all so unique, and the special connection you have with your intuition is just for you. Your intuition is talking to you all the time. Spend a week really paying attention, getting to know yourself and your spirit even more, and figure out how *you* communicate.

Imagine that your intuition is a friend you dearly love. In order to learn from her, you must be openly engaged. This isn't a one-sided relationship, so ask her questions. Get really specific, because the clearer you are in your questions, the clearer the answers will be. And while you're at it, send your intuition some love and appreciation for all that she does for you.

And then, write it down! Neuroscience research concludes that intuitive insights that haven't been captured within 37 seconds will likely never be recalled again. Don't let your beloved wisdom slip through your fingers. I like to always carry a small notebook with me in my purse, because you never know when your intuition is going to pipe up!

Life can get so busy and it is easy to forget to tune in to your intuition. Yes, your intuition will reach out to you, but the biggest insights often come when you are intentionally open to receiving them. Give yourself time every day to check in with yourself. You can take just a few moments each day, perhaps before you eat a meal, before you go to bed, or when you first wake up in the morning, to have a moment of connection. The more consistent you are with showing up for your intuition, the more reliable she will become.

Trusting your intuition comes down to trusting yourself. When you know in your heart, mind, and soul that something is absolute, give yourself the honor of respecting this, even if it means making an uncomfortable shift. Don't be afraid. There is no greater way to love yourself than honoring what you know to be true.

There's one important thing left to do that can support you in locking in these promises and releasing anything that could be holding you back. Remember Mary? Look back to Mary's story of her mom yelling at her while she was playing piano. Do you have a story such as this that made you shrink or feel unworthy? Or do you have someone in your life that you wish you had their love, support, nurturing? Maybe it's more that they trigger your feelings of unworthiness. Sit with yourself and think back to the situation, how old were you? Once you have the answer, write them a letter from that age, let it flow out, let your inner child just write. This may cause a lot of emotions to come up but that's okay, let it flow out of you. Once you've finished writing the story, give yourself some words of encouragement for being so brave to continue moving forward and for doing the work it takes to break free from that cord that's held you from so long ago. You are free. You are seeing the world with different eyes.

The last time I did this what came to me was something that my inner child needed to release from when I was three years old. As I wrote on the paper, it was only scribbles coming out on the other end, I couldn't read a thing, but I could feel the release. I watch my clients release trauma, hurt, old stories, and energy every time they do this and each time they come back lighter, free, empowered, and in full trust.

Trust yourself, trust the age and situation that comes to you. Once you have everything written, take the paper and burn it. You are letting the universe and yourself know that you are no longer available for that treatment, those thoughts or those feelings, and you're ready for a new story.

I love myself
when I have trust
in myself; that is
all I need.

# 15 WAYS TO SPEND EVERY DAY IN LOVE WITH YOU

**1** **Break down old patterns and rediscover a new set of ideals.** By breaking down old patterns and committing yourself to loving you and showing yourself that love, you are giving yourself the most beautiful kind of love and compassion.

**2** **Make four self-love promises to yourself to live by.** Become unavailable for comparison, be kind to yourself, commit to yourself and your dreams first, and trust yourself.

**3** **Get out of the comparison trap.** We often find ourselves comparing ourselves to others and what they have, and while this is normal, we are doing more harm to ourselves than we are helping. Remember, you are running your own race, and everything will come to you in due time.

**4** **Remember that social media doesn't show the whole picture.** People post what they want you to see and while it may seem like all these influencers have it all, there is a story behind every picture.

**5** **Be authentically yourself.** When you are authentically you, you are setting yourself free to express your truth.

**6** **Be aware of your comparison habits and find the root of your comparison habits.** Figure out what it is that you are comparing and why. Once you know why, you can take the time to unpack your feelings and work to come from a place of love instead of hate.

**7** **Redirect comparison back to you.** Practice unlearning comparison habits by letting go of any comparison thoughts and focusing on you. Think something positive about yourself and know that what is meant for you will make its way to you.

**8** **Use the four A's (page 69) to stop yourself from falling into the comparison trap.** Become aware of your thoughts, accept that they are there, create positive affirmations, and take action toward what you desire.

**9** **Let go of negative self-talk.** Confront negative thoughts as they arise and declare a new thought. Practice flipping your thoughts from negative to positive often.

**10** **Say "no" more often.** Sometimes, we can find ourselves saying "yes" to things that drain our energy and do us more harm than good. This will be hard to do, especially when we say "no" to the people we care about, but if something is not doing you good, then "no" is the right answer. Being kind to yourself is showing up for you. No need for explanations.

**11** **Track your calendar.** Look at your calendar and pick out the things that are making you feel bad or are draining you that are not important, and start replacing those things with stuff you enjoy doing.

**12** **Figure out what you want.** Spend time writing down your goals, dreams, and desires and start prioritizing things in your calendar that lead you closer to them.

**13** **Trust yourself.** Listen to your intuition. It will always steer you in the right direction.

**14** **Let go of fear.** We often find ourselves not taking risks or not taking action toward what we want out of fear of failing at it, but by doing that, we are cutting chances and opportunities out of our lives. Keep going through the fear and do the thing you want to do anyway. When you do that, you will see that things will turn out okay. Even if you fail at it, it will serve as a lesson for the next time.

**15** **Be brave.** Trust your intuition and drown out the self-limiting beliefs that try to take over. Your intuition is your friend and it will be there for you always.

## Homework: Promise School

We learn all about keeping promises to others but what about keeping promises to ourselves? Your word and promise to you means something, and when you don't keep it you suffer inside. Here is the thing about promises: in order to make one that you can truly keep, you must tune in to you. You must know yourself and be in the constant practice of asking yourself what's going on inside. When you are keeping up with yourself and cultivating your relationship to self it will become rare that you would ever break a promise, because when you make them, you will be making them from your highest self. A woman who loves herself keeps her promises to herself.

Follow the steps in the exercise below to help you keep promises to yourself.

**Step 1: Stay in touch.** For the next week, set a timer on your phone every couple of hours. Have the reminder be a check-in. When the timer goes off, place your hand on your heart, close your eyes, and check in. Ask yourself:

- Is there anything I need at this moment?
- Is there anything that I want me to know?
- What can I do for myself right now?

You'll get the answers, and as you do this more and more, you will get them clearer and clearer. When you get the answers, honor them. This practice is giving yourself time and space to listen, and when you then honor those answers with an action that fills you up, you let yourself know that you are safe, that you can trust, and your confidence and love for yourself will start to soar.

**Step 2: Confess your love in the mirror.**
Let's try an experiment! Once a day for twenty-one days look at yourself in the mirror. Stare into your beautiful eyes and smile. Look at yourself for 2 minutes a day and use your eyes to express love to yourself. Smile, admire, express. For 1 minute, do this in complete silence, and when you feel called, talk to yourself. Let the words flow out: "I love me. I'm beautiful. I'm an amazing queen. I can do this. I was meant for this. I have an amazing life. I like how much I shine." Keep a journal of the first few days to record your thoughts about this experiment and what comes up for you, and then do the same the last few days of the experiment. After twenty-one days, read both sections; you may be surprised at the results and will be grateful you kept a record of it!

**Step 3: Practice.** There's no better way to have something stick than to practice it. During the twenty-one days of mirror work, keep a promise list. Every day, write one thing on your list that you promise to do for yourself. Commit each day to doing that *one* thing no matter what happens and schedule it in as a priority in your day so that you set yourself up for success. This will cultivate unwavering commitment inside yourself and show you how that commitment to yourself can be life altering. You do not need to make these big things; they can be small. In fact, I suggest starting smaller. Here are some examples:

- Drinking eight glasses of water a day
- Going for a walk
- Journaling
- Taking a 5-minute break of silence
- Laughing

**Higher Love Level:** Reward yourself after the twenty-one days. Literally have a celebration dinner, buy yourself something, or do an at-home spa day. Show your body that not only can it count on you, but also that you will reward yourself. Celebration is a huge part of living a high-vibe lifestyle.

> **Love yourself through it all and keep falling in love with all parts of you.**

# I SHINE
# MY LIGHT

# Chapter 4

# MADE FOR SELF-CARE

**EARLIER WE POKED** a few holes in the idea that self-care is self-indulgent, or that it doesn't necessarily have anything to do with "treating yourself." First, let me remind you that self-care is a *necessity.* It's not a treat or a special occasion or something you do every once in a while. Self-care is something you do every day, and it's as important as breathing and drinking water.

Self-care is how you show yourself love. Demonstrating love is important in all our relationships, whether it's with our partners, our children, our parents, our siblings, or our friends, and we do it in so many different ways. We tell them we love them, yes, but we also do the dishes when it isn't our turn because we know they've had a long day. We pack special treats in their lunch boxes. We let them tell us the same story over and over and laugh like it's the first time. We call them up out of the blue just because we were thinking about them. The little things we do for the people we love show them how much we love them. Shouldn't we do the same for ourselves?

By this point, you get it—your relationship with yourself is the most important relationship you've got. Period. So, you'd better make sure you take care of it, putting just as much attention on it as any other relationship—maybe even more! You can't just love yourself. You've got to show it.

Self-care is an attitude, a standard, and an action that lets your soul know you are a priority and you are ready to receive an extraordinary life. Self-care happens when you know you are giving yourself all the love in the world, when you protect your peace, appreciate your body, and treat your time as the precious thing that it is.

When you've got self-care going on, you won't be bothered with made-up ideas of perfection. It is when we aren't loving ourselves or giving ourselves self-care that we obsess over things that are not real, like society's ideas of how we ought to be in the world. Here's the thing about perfection: it's only real when it's your own and when it comes from a place of complete appreciation, acceptance, gratitude, and pure love for all that is you. It's when you decide to believe that you are a perfect being that is growing and evolving and everything is working out as it should.

But what exactly does that mean? It means you are the only one who can create perfection in you, and the only way to do that is by knowing and accepting all parts of you, knowing your path and honoring every cell inside of you because you are the perfect you. You are because you say you are. You're the only one to compare yourself to.

**You are the only one that is on your path every step of the way.**

Tell yourself you are the perfect you and that you promise to do the things that honor, cherish, and continue to evolve that perfection that only you can have.

You are an incredible gift in the world. There is only one you and you serve a magical purpose on this planet. Whether or not you believe this, it is a miracle that you are here. Everything needed to align a certain way to produce the beautiful person you see in the mirror every day.

Because every detail and step is individually yours, the way you take care of yourself is a discovery that only you can decide. You will constantly be changing the things you do to show yourself love because you are someone who will be constantly evolving. Did you know that every seven to ten years, you are made up of an entirely new set of cells…yep, you physically become a whole new person! So, what is to stop you from emotionally becoming a new person too? The goal is to look back a week from now, a month from now, a year from now, and smile because you don't recognize yourself anymore because you have evolved beyond words. When you are doing the things that fill you up and create peace, joy, and support in your body, mind, and soul, you are treasuring the absolute beautiful creation that is you.

You deserve to feel seen, supported, loved, and cherished. The way you receive this is by first doing it for yourself. You are the most important person that your highest self, your soul, and your heart needs. Love from you creates the power to do anything that you could possibly ever dream of doing. The love from you creates the miracles that your inner voice knows are possible. Again, the way you show your love for yourself depends on *you*. You don't show your love for everyone in your life in exactly the same way, so why would anyone think that self-care looks the same for everyone? Be curious about discovering your self-care language and the things you feel in your body. Your body and soul will let you know what it needs, craves, and feels. You just need to give yourself a break and listen.

There are several different types of self-care, all are important, but some are needed more often. What self-care exactly looks like depends on you! It's not about forcing yourself to give yourself self-care but more about figuring out the kind that is best for you. If there is a certain type of self-care ritual that just doesn't do it for you, awesome! Figure out what does because your care will bring you so many answers and will support you in every area of your life.

There's a difference between not liking one ritual and just not doing it because you are being lazy, stuck, or unwilling to get out of your comfort zone. Remember that "just fine" is not what you are on this planet for, you are here for the ultimate level of love and joy. One of the most nurturing things you can do for yourself is get truly committed to your self-care game and learn what your inner and outer body, soul, and mind need to feel your best. Self-care is restorative, magical, nurturing, and improves your self-worth.

Here are some of the different types of self-care that are crucial to focus on:

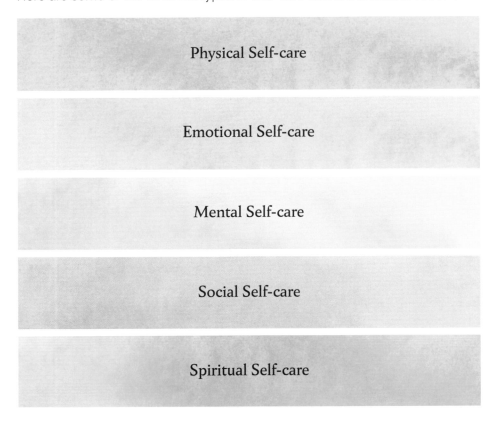

Physical Self-care

Emotional Self-care

Mental Self-care

Social Self-care

Spiritual Self-care

**Physical Self-care** is taking care of your physical body, your health, your diet, eating foods that are good for you, knowing what your body responds negatively to and positively to, moving your body, staying hydrated, walking, and taking care of your sleep routines. When you are practicing physical self-care you are taking care of the beautiful body that was gifted to you, the vessel that allows you to be here on this planet. When you do things to physically take care of yourself, you are restoring the gift that the universe gave to you so that you could love your life and fulfill your purpose while moving throughout your days.

**Emotional Self-care** is all about your inner well-being. It is when you are taking the care to acknowledge your inner world, your feelings, your desire, and your inner self. Much of what we are talking about in this book is about emotional self-care, for when you are taking care of yourself emotionally, you are loving yourself. Emotional self-care allows you to get to know the inner you.

It is the inner work you do when you listen to your emotions, whether it's anger, sadness, or joy, you are caring for yourself when you step away from the noise and sit down with your feelings and get to know them. Once you know what you really feel, not only does self-acceptance start to manifest, but also you'll know exactly what negative emotions and behaviors you want to reprogram. Your emotional self-care is reflected by the frequency you vibe at.

**Mental Self-care** is much of each self-care area combined, as the way you are taking care yourself can impact your mental health and well-being. Taking care of yourself physically and emotionally impacts your mental health. Keeping your mind sharp, engaged, learning new things, and diving in to create avenues will improve and keep you on your game to nourish your mind.

**Social Self-care** is so important, and many times it can get overlooked. It is not only about being around people but also being around the right people for you. We talk about this so much throughout each chapter because this has a huge impact on you personally. Because in today's world, "success" and social media are so in our face it's easy to forget about the right type of social self-care for you. You might be interacting on social media and texting with people, but this isn't taking care of the parts of you that need a deeper, more nurturing connection. Text messages and no other interaction is not taking care of your social needs. Don't get me wrong, I am a huge advocate for texting, but I make it a priority to have in-person connections and have face-to-face calls. The more you do this, the better your people and social skills will be. Because your inner self can feel the level of connection you have with others, your relationships will impact your life in every way. Also, from a law of attraction standpoint, the more connected you are with people, the more you are giving to them and supporting them, the more you feel supported and the higher frequency you will be.

**Spiritual Self-care** is pure heaven. It allows you to tap into your highest self, connect to nature, listen to your soul, and receive messages from the universe. Practices like journaling, meditation, prayer, and self-development connect you to a higher purpose, a higher being, your highest self, and cause a radiant light from inside of you to shine outward. Regardless of your religious beliefs, when you are creating space to connect to something greater than you, you are able to feel a higher energy and power and tap deep into your own true self. Let's discover what works best for you and build a road map through this chapter together!

# FIGURING OUT YOUR LOVE LANGUAGE FOR YOUR SELF-CARE NEEDS

**SELF-CARE MEANS SO** many different things and figuring out what it means for you starts with looking at what you need in your relationship with yourself. What's your personal love language? If you aren't familiar with love languages, these are means by which you give and receive love. According to Dr. Gary Chapman, there are five love languages: physical touch, acts of service, words of affirmation, gifts, and quality time. While this concept is often referenced in relation to how we give and receive love to other people, it can also be applied to loving ourselves.

Let's dive in a little bit to your self-love language and what type of self-care you need most! If you know that you are someone who thrives off **physical touch**, then self-care that is made for you specifically includes things that make your body feel good and that take care of your physical well-being. Massages, spa days, movement, soft blankets, pillows, hugging, and things that get into your body.

If you are someone who loves **acts of service** it's important that you do things for yourself, make plans, and create self-care environments for yourself. Going to therapy, having a life coach, cleaning, scheduling, going out with friends, treating yourself to a date that is planned out in advance, and making plans for yourself will really ignite your self-care and feelings of being cared for.

Throughout these chapters, you will be hearing how important the words you say to yourself are. If you identify in love with **words of affirmation**, then a self-care practice of doubling down on the words you say to yourself is vital. Pep talks and encouragement are going to be important for you in your self-care. Mantras and having a list of daily affirmations that you recite will be life altering for you. Give yourself the words and compliments that you long to receive.

If you are filled with love when a significant other gives you a thoughtful **gift**, treat yourself to something special on occasion. Part of self-care is also doing the things needed to get back into your feminine power and being open to receiving gifts, support, love, help, compliments, and so on. If you love to receive presents, something that is important for you to create for yourself in your self-care practices is treating yourself, not just pampering yourself but also doing things that make you happy. You can do things like go on trips, wear comfy clothes, and spend the whole day journaling. Invest in yourself with things that will further your education, self-development, and well-being.

If you feel the most love when someone spends **quality time** with you, gift yourself an evening of quality time with only you. Take yourself on a date or stay in and give yourself a face mask treatment while you listen to your favorite playlist. We often forget that spending time with ourselves is needed, it's part of developing a relationship with yourself and also part of taking care of yourself. Spending time with you is a part of your mental and spiritual self-care, and if you are someone who connects to those you spend quality time with, you must set aside quality time even more so with yourself. Quality time for you looks like *alone* time. Meditation is key for quality time and spiritual connection. The act of relaxing is also part of spending quality time with yourself. Planning spontaneous and unplanned dates for yourself is another way to spend quality time with yourself.

**Just like we have certain things that connect us to others, part of our self-care is to do the things that connect us to ourselves and tailoring your self-care to you is a great way to create peace, joy, and well-being inside of you.**

Pampering is important in praising yourself, and it's fun! It often seems like we think self-care is limited to a very short menu. That's all we get to order, and oftentimes, there's nothing on there we really want. Not everyone likes taking bubble baths!

To figure out what counts as self-care for *you*, think about the things you do to rid yourself of negative energy. You might not even realize you're doing them! Imagine yourself in a stressful situation, the kind of thing that comes up pretty often, like being stuck in traffic or getting into an argument with a coworker. Feel that experience in your body. You may notice your muscles starting to tense up just from the memory.

Okay, shake it off. Literally shake it off! Now think about it—what do you do after those situations? When you're sitting in traffic, do you queue up your favorite jam? Do you take a minute to list off what you are grateful for?

Do you calm yourself down? When you finally get where you're going, do you get yourself a cup of tea or a glass of ice water and take a minute so that you can be your best self for what you're about to step into next? When you're walking away from an argument, do you go find your friend who's always good for a laugh? Do you reach for one of your values? Or have you been doing some more unhealthy things, like grabbing the phone to gossip or spending the week complaining about every single thing that happened? This only creates more anxiety in your body. By doing things to bring up the stress, pain, or event over again, your body is left with a lower frequency, and it really needs you to refresh and level up the frequency.

What if you decide after these types of experiences that you're worth it and are going to do something to support your mind and body to experience joy or peace and have its back by choosing not to put it through the ringer, again? Imagine your body as a child that had a tantrum or needs love after a traumatic event. Give it something positive to get the energy out and distract it with love and joy. Do not put it through the situation over again by neglecting the self-care it needs. For instance, when you have an argument or are upset about something, get it out, call someone to vent to, or write it out, and then choose to triple down on things that fill you up. Follow the steps below to practice more self-care daily.

**STEP 1**    Get it out and then choose to leave it so that you can do what you need to step into the higher frequency.

**STEP 2**    Fill yourself with things that feed your soul, that ignite joy, not things that numb the feeling.

**STEP 3**    Remind yourself that you have your own back and that is enough. We need to hear that from the person we are closest to: ourselves.

You can have your own back through self-care in so many ways.

I love myself when
I allow myself to feel
cherished. I am a
masterpiece, a goddess,
an empress, a queen.

# WHEN WE NEED SELF-CARE MOST

**LOVING YOURSELF IS** the number one asset to having anything you want in life. You may or may not know this, but it's because you are your biggest asset. And your self-care is a part of how you show love to yourself, have your own back, nurture, and grow with your soul throughout your journey and this human experience. Love, nourish, and take care of your asset! Life experiences, heartache, loss, and hurt will take you away from caring for yourself, and it is those times when you need to care for yourself the most. Always advocate for self-care. Take care of yourself as the vessel because it is the container for your life.

Think about someone you care so much about—maybe it's a friend, a family member, your partner, or your child. If they were lying on the ground, needing help, hurting, completely undone, would you walk away from them or would you do anything you possibly could to soothe them in that moment? I am guessing that you would do anything you could to soothe them. Then why would you not do the same for yourself?

When you are down, low, sad, or feeling rejected, do you abandon your self-care routine? When it gets tough and when you need love the most, do you treat yourself with kindness? Do you drop everything and run to your own rescue, giving yourself anything that you could possibly need?

It takes some thought to figure out how to show up for yourself when *you* are the one hurting. And we hurt in so many different ways throughout our lives. The following sections cover some common wounds we all face at some point, along with some tips for self-care, to show yourself love when you need it most.

# REJECTION

**REJECTION IS A PAINFUL** feeling. It can feel like you're not included, like you've failed, or like there's something wrong with you, and all of that is hard to take. No matter how often we feel rejected, it doesn't seem to get any easier. We have this experience over and over—all of us do, including me! And it always hurts just as much as it did the first time. We never get used to it.

Why is that? Rejection is something we all experience, but it's also something we never talk about. We curl in around this painful feeling, protecting it, not letting anyone else see that we're feeling it. We run away from it or pretend it didn't happen and we do everything in our power to prevent it from ever happening again.

I'm going to hit you with something: you can't run away from rejection. You will experience that feeling again. But here's what you need to know: rejection is simply life's way of showing you that something is not meant for you. This thing you wanted, it's not for you to experience. There's something better out there, just waiting for you.

Rejection is a gift.

It's a pretty awful-feeling gift, but it's necessary.

You can't change the way rejection feels in your body, but you can change the meaning you make of it. Rather than deciding that your rejection means that something is wrong *with you*, consider that something about the thing you wanted is wrong *for you*. Embrace your experience of that rejection and look at it as if it were a compass, pointing you toward something that is better for you.

**We are never truly rejected; we are simply redirected.**

It does take some self-care to get ourselves to that point. After all, rejection still hurts, even if we accept that it's for the best! You can love yourself through your rejection by doing things for yourself, such as journaling it out. Most importantly, when it comes to rejection, your response must be to give yourself some major positive self-talk and encouragement, immediately. Remind yourself that in every situation, no matter what, nothing is ever personal, that your viewpoint of someone's actions being a rejection of you has nothing to do with you and everything to do with them. You quite literally do not know what is behind it or what their motives or own fears are.

When you feel and experience rejection, you absolutely get to vent it out and do what you need to release it, but if you immediately show up for yourself and talk yourself through the emotion, you will not be so taken down by the gut-wrenching feeling that rejection can bring. Take the time to work through it, rather than running from it or simply spinning out in the emotional pain of the rejection over and over again. You are worthy of the time and effort it takes to dive in and explore this. Here are some questions you can ask yourself:

What was it that I thought I wanted?

What happened? Why do I feel rejected?

What does this mean?
What does this redirection tell me about what I truly want?

Where is my compass pointing now?

Another tool to support yourself through this is to think back on a situation in the past when you felt rejected. What did you find out later that reminded you that you were either not rejected or that it was actually a blessing in disguise? For me, breakups have served as this reminder that someone better for me or truly meant for my highest good was to come. I have also had so much rejection in the industry that I am in, as I am sure you have experienced in your career or in anything that has competition. For me, in those times, it has always turned out that either something better was around the corner or that there was something behind the scenes that had nothing to do with me. These are the things I remind myself of when "rejection" hits. What has it been like for you? In these moments, it is crucial to remind yourself of these experiences in the past that ended up not being as they seemed or that guided you to something better. Make a list of all the times something great came from a rejection to refer back to, grab your list when you need it, and give yourself some serious love through your words and reminders.

# JEALOUSY

**SOMETIMES IT FEELS** like all we do every day is compare ourselves to others, which leads to not only a question of worthiness in ourselves, but also a spark of jealousy. Social media is definitely a huge part of this. We scroll through and see what our friends are doing, what someone we admire is doing, and inevitably we start to feel bad about ourselves…we become jealous. That friend has a third book coming out. That former colleague just got *another* promotion. That woman just married someone she just met, and you are not even engaged yet! Insert, shame, fear, worry, and jealousy. This may send you into a spiral of jealousy, blinding you and altering your own perception of reality. And all of this comparison and jealous behavior creates nothing fun. In fact, according to research, jealousy results in emotional instability, depression, anxiety, and lack of security.

I love myself
when I choose a new
direction and believe
that there's something
better coming
for me.

The thing about comparing ourselves with others is that it's completely natural. According to some psychological studies, as much as 10 percent of our thoughts involve comparisons of some kind. It's something we do when we are simply trying to figure out who we are and how to be in the world. We are taught from a very young age that comparison is a good thing. "Look at Sally! She's using a spoon! You can use a spoon, too!" Unfortunately, this is where jealousy comes from and where it starts.

We use other people as models to show us how to do things, and to help us figure out the right or wrong thing to do in any given situation. Comparison is a compass that helps us understand how to be in the world. It's also dangerous. It sets us on a path where we can end up unable to fully embody our true selves. Every step we take down jealousy street takes us further and further away from ourselves, until we lose our inner knowing. We end up listening only to others and ignoring our own voice. The danger with jealousy is that we often only compare ourselves to paragons, or the perfect example of a desired characteristic. For example, you may think you have a less successful career than others, but that is because when making this observation, you compare yourself only to the most successful people you know. In large part, how we react to comparison is dependent upon who we compare ourselves to. If you can recognize this bias thought, you can make more realistic and motivational observations.

So, how do we break free from jealousy? It starts with identifying the root of the behavior. This may sound harsh, but your jealousy likely stems from your greatest insecurity. Studies have found that jealousy is directly correlated to lower levels of self-esteem. Think about it, whatever you want to improve most in your life, is likely what you are most envious of in other people.

When you find yourself feeling jealous, get intentional and sift through the thoughts coming up. Consider what the aspect of jealousy, be it a friend's promotion or a picture of a beautifully fit influencer, relates to in your personal life. Perhaps you were told you weren't good at math, so you never felt smart enough to get that promotion, or maybe you struggled with your weight as a teenager and are triggered by being made fun of for your size. The more you can connect your jealous emotion to a past event, the easier it becomes to release the envious emotion.

The more you can focus on feeling strong and secure in yourself, the less jealous you will become. Every one of us, even famous people, are full of what others may view as flaws and limitations. This is why it is beyond important to practice self-compassion in the face of jealousy and stand up to your own inner critic.

The moment I feel a jealous tingle coming on, I take a deep breath, and say to myself one thing I love about who I am. I also send that person love, even and especially when it feels the most difficult. This way I am able to send my brain a different message, while at the same time show up for my body's reactions and let the universe know that that's something I am available for. And from here, I can observe what I admire in the other person or situation with awe and inspiration.

When you feel jealousy, it leads to you shaming another person or shaming something they have, and this sends a signal to the universe that you don't like this "thing" you're jealous of, therefore you push that "thing" further away from you. This is why jealousy hurts you, not just the person you feel jealous of. When you are jealous, recognize it, dive into it, and if the reason you are jealous is because you want to experience or have what this person has, then send them love, internally congratulate them. Yes, it is hard, but it will support you in having fewer and fewer feelings of jealousy. It will also signal to the universe that you are ready for that experience or thing but in the way it is meant for you. This immediately shifts your mind from a negative place into a more positive, inspired place.

**Instead of focusing on not being jealous, focus on getting back into alignment.**

The self-care process of getting back into alignment can mean doing the things you love! If you have a hobby you enjoy, like painting, cooking, or writing, spend some time doing that. The things that light us up are an antidote to jealousy. If you're feeling happy and fulfilled, you can explore comparison the way it's meant to be used—as a way of checking in with yourself.

If you scroll through social media and see a friend who has just bought a new house, you can be happy for her and not feel envious of her. You can think, "That's cool that she has that. Do I desire to have that?" If your answer is "yes," you create a plan to manifest this desire and you decide to focus on bringing that into your life rather than hating on those who have it or bringing yourself down for not having those things quite yet, therefore prolonging and preventing it from happening even more. If your answer is "no," then you realize it's not something you are interested in right now or maybe even ever. This check-in can help you figure out how to move forward in life while still staying in alignment with who you are and what you want. Whenever you're hit with a painful jealous moment, immediately go do something that brings you joy. Something fun, something you're proud of—something that gets you back to you.

You will experience jealousy at various points in your life and that is okay. The important thing is that you redirect your focus on finding out why you're feeling this way. Find the root of the cause and then take the time to heal that part of you. Once you align the part of you that needs healing, you'll be able to see things from a place of abundance instead of a place of lack. The universe will return to you what you put out, so if you reach from a place of abundance, you will be more open to receiving what it is that you desire.

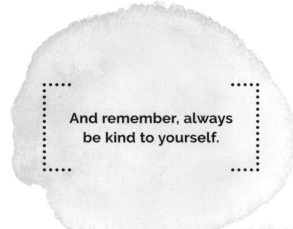

And remember, always be kind to yourself.

I love myself
when I have fun, look
for ways to express my
true genius, and shine
my inner light.

# BETRAYAL

**BETRAYAL IS ONE** of the lowest-vibrational hurtful experiences we can have. We feel it in our hearts, weighing us down, and in the moment, it can feel like the most painful experience ever. And like everything else on this list, it's inevitable. We can never fully protect ourselves from being hurt by others, and if we try, we simply end up cutting ourselves off from life and blocking the blessing waiting for us.

Hurt people hurt people. Sometimes they hurt us on purpose, and sometimes it's by accident, but every single person has caused someone else pain. You, too, have hurt people, even when you didn't mean to. And yet, there are times when we are hurt by someone and it feels unbearable—and that's when pain turns into betrayal. We simply never saw it coming, and we shift into comparison, that potentially dangerous way of approaching the world. We try to put ourselves in their shoes, and we think, "I would never do that. I would never cheat. I would never say that, I would never (fill in the blank)."

But the thing is, we can never actually know another person's experience. We can only ever know our own experiences, and more importantly, our own sense of self-worth and self-love. If someone is feeling worthless, they often do things to prove that they are, in fact, not worthy of our love. It doesn't make it okay, and it definitely still hurts, but there is nothing to be gained from trying to compare our choices with theirs. Betrayal and rejection live in the same neighborhood and many times we can judge our own self-worth based on being betrayed or rejected. The irrational thoughts can creep in: "Well, if I was pretty enough, then they wouldn't have cheated" or "If I was good enough, I would have been picked."

The reason betrayal hurts is because of the meaning we give it. We ask ourselves why; we try to understand how they could do this when we gave so much to them and did so much for them. The truth is, their betrayal has little to do with you, and the more time and energy you spend trying to figure out *why* is just more energy that you are giving to them.

> **Rather than focusing on the pain of their betrayal, focus on yourself.**

Don't give in to the temptation to close off your heart. Instead, the thing to do is to remain open and pour so much love into your heart. The first thing that you must do is let yourself feel the hurt rather than push it away, because the sooner you allow yourself to feel and process, the sooner you will heal. Let yourself feel the pain, surround yourself with a support system, triple down on your self-care, and spend even more time with yourself. The first thing many people do is go into avoidance; they stay angry and bitter, but they run directly out to do the things that are fleeting, the hydronic happiness. The more loved you are, the more you are going to be able to recognize toxic relationships and stay away from them. The more self-love you have to give, the more attuned you will be to what you need. You'll also be more aware of the energy around you, and the energy coming off of someone. You'll be able to see whether this person is someone you want to be around.

We can learn to avoid these people and prevent ourselves from seeking them out by making sure that we are as free from hurt as we can be. Our self-love can fill our hearts so that we aren't reaching so hard for love from others. We are all that we truly need, and whatever else we receive from those who love us is just an amazing bonus.

We cannot control what other people do. We cannot protect ourselves from them. But if you keep an open heart and work on yourself, then there will be nothing to protect.

When betrayal does hit, it takes time to recover. So often we see people, either those who betray or who have been betrayed (and make no mistake—both people in that situation are hurting, because both of them are human), and they act as if nothing happened. Just like rejection, we want to run away from it and pretend it doesn't exist. That simply doesn't work. If you go on without processing your betrayal, you might seem fine on the outside, even to yourself, but you'll end up carrying that pain within you for years, perhaps even for the rest of your life.

> **Time and reflection heal betrayal.**

I love myself when
I am honest with myself.
I love every cell in my body.
I give thanks to myself
and attract health, joy, and
abundance when I do
things that feed my soul.

Self-care in this case means giving yourself the space to realize what happened, accept it, and recover from it. Spend a week, two weeks, a month really feeling those feelings, so you don't carry them. You will get over your betrayal sooner if you let yourself experience it and feel it.

To properly begin to process, you must get very honest with yourself and say what happened out loud. Many times, because it feels so painful and we associate rejection or betrayal unconsciously with something being wrong with us, we do not fully admit to ourselves or others that this was done to us, for fear that it would say something about our worth. To process any betrayal, you must be brutally honest with yourself about the facts of what was done. Once you give yourself the gift to feel the pain and be completely honest with what happened, without trying to justify or leave parts out, you will be able to move through it faster because you are moving through what is, not what you have decided to make up about it. You will begin to have epiphanies of signs that you missed in the situation (use these as lessons and reminders to trust your intuition; do not use them to get further down on yourself). Embrace this experience as best you can to grow further into your power. Use this betrayal as a guiding point, as a lesson, as something to better yourself.

# SELF-DOUBT

**WE ALL EXPERIENCE** self-doubt. I experience it. I bet you even the most famous people experience it. It is just another part of life. Self-doubt is our mind's way of trying to protect us from failure. Trying something new is scary—it's a risk, and the mind is incredibly risk-averse. The mind feels safe in what it knows, and it would far rather that you stay exactly where you are, in what you know, so that you remain safe.

When your heart starts asking you for something more, your mind starts getting worried. It says, "Whoa, whoa, whoa, put on the brakes there! This terrible thing might happen! Or that one!" And your mind is right—things might not work out exactly as you wish (though it probably won't be as terrible as your mind claims it will). But if something matters to you, your heart is willing to take that risk . . . and that's when your mind pulls out its secret weapon.

Self-doubt is a powerful tool the mind uses to protect you from risk. It feels true because it goes right to our most vulnerable, tender fears and beliefs about ourselves.

But just because something feels true doesn't mean it is true.

So how do you drown out that protective voice? We all move through different stages of self-doubt. If we're just at the beginning of our journey of self-work, or if we've been hit with a bunch of obstacles and challenges, that voice of self-doubt can be pretty loud. It can be so loud, in fact, that we don't even recognize it for what it is and think that we're listening to the voice of logic, of reason, of practicality.

Self-doubt is none of those things. The first step to quieting your self-doubt is to become aware of it. Making a habit of speaking kindly to yourself will definitely help! Once you begin to recognize self-doubt for what it is—a protective mechanism—you can begin to reply to it. You can say, "I know you're trying to help, but you're actually just causing me pain and making things more difficult, and I'm not available for that."

Saying "no" to self-doubt and negative self-talk is just the same as saying "no" to anything else that isn't serving you.

But like I said, self-doubt comes up for everyone. Even if you've been working on yourself for years and years and you're successful and amazing and obviously can do anything you set your mind to—self-doubt will still show up. It comes when you're ready to level up, to step into a bigger game. It comes when you haven't been giving yourself enough space to hear your true internal voice. And sometimes, it will even just appear at random! You'll be going along, feeling good, and then, wham! You get hit with self-doubt.

It's okay. It happens, and it doesn't have to mean anything. The key, again, is to remember what self-doubt is, and what it isn't.

**Self-doubt is a way for your mind to protect you. That doesn't make it true.**

I love myself
when I listen to
my heart.

Here's how you know it's not true: when you ignore self-doubt and do it anyway. Go after exactly what you want, despite the self-doubt, and prove your protective mind wrong! Then you'll get to say, "Okay, wow, that wasn't the truth at all," and you'll have proof for next time. Trust me, the more you prove your self-doubt wrong, the easier it becomes to shush it the next time it pipes up.

And when you do get caught in a loop of self-doubt, double down on your self-care. Self-care trains us to maintain unwavering belief in ourselves. The best form of self-care for self-doubt is monitoring your self-talk. Negative self-talk goes hand in hand with self-doubt, and you can drown it out by intentionally practicing positive self-talk.

When you experience self-doubt, speak aloud these affirmations: *I have all that I need, and I am all that I need. I trust myself. I am worthy of my dreams.*

# SADNESS

**SADNESS COMES IN** two forms: it can occur when you've gone through a painful experience, like a breakup or a death. And it can also come when you have been ignoring yourself, and not giving yourself the love you need and deserve. We experience a deep, heavy feeling, and it can feel impossible to carry, and yet we can't imagine that we will ever be without it.

> **The thing about sadness is that it isn't the illness itself, it's the symptom. And like a fever, it's a symptom that is actively working to help you heal.**

Sadness is your indicator that you are hurting, and if you ignore it, you will only feel worse and worse. Sadness is the thing we must go through in order to heal. There is so much beauty and magic in giving yourself the space to feel sadness and allowing it to heal you. It may feel like you will never be without sadness, particularly if you're mourning a deep loss, but your sadness will change, I promise. You will never be without the recognition of the loss and what it means, but you don't need to hold it within you, poisoning you. You can allow it to heal and find its place in acceptance.

In order to do this, you must give yourself permission to feel your sadness. Ignoring this feeling doesn't change how you feel, so embrace it. Feel it. Pay attention to it. If you don't, it will just get stuck inside you. Think about how you shake a bottle and then when you open it, it explodes. That's what will happen if you don't immediately give your sadness the care it needs.

Remember the phrase "hurt people hurt people"? You've been hurt by others who didn't deal with their pain. It's your responsibility, your work, to be aware of your feelings and take care of them. You don't want to get to the point where your sadness causes you to harm yourself or others. It's so much easier, and better, to deal with your feelings early, when you first experience them, rather than letting them poison you, and then having to go through a full detox.

Don't rush through the process of caring for your sadness. It takes time. Cry it out and let your body process it. If your sadness gets to be too much for you, it's all right to ask for help. Part of self-care is getting help and knowing when sadness is beginning to overwhelm you and your life.

> **Your sadness is an indicator light, and it will let you know the self-care you need.**

Treat yourself the way you would treat someone you love when they are hurting. Hold yourself, be gentle with yourself. Remind yourself that everything will get better.

I love myself
when I take the
time to heal.

# REGRET

**REGRET IS A STAGE** past sadness. Sadness is out of our control; we are sad most times about something we can't do anything about. Regret is painful because it's something we *did* have control over. With other challenging emotions, we can say, "This wasn't in my control; this isn't mine." But regret *is* ours to carry. We often carry this feeling of regret into the future. And this lingering regret may be linked to what part of the brain mediates the feeling of remorse: the medial orbitofrontal cortex, the part of the brain that is also involved in the process of decision-making. So later down the road when faced with a similar situation, we may make a decision rooted in the regret we still feel.

I recently went through this.

Years ago, I was preparing for one of my first live events. I had to place bids and shop around for a location to support the big day. I knew I was confirmed to have two hundred women attend but wasn't sure if more would sign up in time to warrant a larger space. In the moment, I thought not too many more would sign up, and I went with the smaller venue. Girl, let me tell you, I regretted that decision, because fifty more women ended up signing up! Luckily, the location was able to swiftly give me a larger space and it all worked out, but moving forward, I have never forgotten that experience and always prepare above and beyond and hold the vision for greatness.

Sometimes regret is something you could have done and didn't, and sometimes it's something you did do and wish you hadn't. We say something we shouldn't have or make a choice that hurts someone. A lot of times, more often than we realize, we can ease regret by making amends, and that's important.

But that's not all there is to it.

> **Regret is important, and we should never push it away. It's a gift to help us do better next time.**

You can reverse engineer why you were so angry and said something you wish you could take back—this kind of understanding can help you prevent it from happening again. For me, my regret taught me that I am extremely powerful. My intuition *knows*, and every time I ignore it, something I don't like will pop up to push me back to listening to my intuition. Regret is a signal that there is something that needs to be tweaked, that needs our attention.

Regret requires self-forgiveness. We may think forgiving others is difficult, and it is, but forgiving ourselves is the hardest of all. But know this: regret is telling you that you are not perfect. You made a mistake; we all do. Self-forgiveness requires acknowledging the mistake, learning from it, and asking how you are different now, how you have changed since making this decision that you now regret. You can't take back your choice, but you can learn from it.

Self-care for regret looks a little different from other kinds of self-care. You're not going to be able to just take a soothing bath and suddenly feel better, but doing something to ground yourself—like getting outside, being in nature, breathing deeply—will be a step that builds. In this instance, regret *is* self-care. It's proving to yourself that you care enough to do the necessary work on yourself. That said, if taking a walk will ground you, and taking a bath will soothe you, do that—it's important to do everything, because the little things add up just as much as the bigger things!

Through regret you can learn more about yourself. If you regret something, you always learn something. You learn what you do not want to be doing to others or yourself. You learn what you will do differently next time. Regret sucks. Recently my husband and I took a lesson from regret. We were celebrating our anniversary and looking back on our last ten years together, and we realized how fast time goes by. We celebrated the amazing moments and our journey. We got super honest about the times we allowed anger, pressure, or any other low vibe take over for far too long. We both realized there was a good two years that we spent most days in stress, striving for business success, putting that first and forgetting to have fun. We hadn't spent as much time with our friends, ourselves, and we missed out on key moments. As we talked, we were both filled up with regret and the painful feeling of knowing that we could very well let this go on forever—and many people do.

We will never get that time back, but we will also always be doing our best not to take time for granted. There is a reason that so many people at the end of their life report their top regret for not living the life they truly wanted. Another regret that is widely shared is not spending present time with the ones they loved or with themselves. Regret is tough because it's something that we actually have control over. You cannot regret something someone else does, you can only regret something that you did or did not do. As you commit to yourself more and more and listen to your inner voice you will have less and less regret in your life.

Do whatever is necessary to get the space you need to dive into this work. When you feel regret, come back to this chapter and dive into the feeling. What's behind it? What will you declare that you will do differently next time?

**You love yourself enough for this. You love yourself enough to not just beat yourself up over it, but to listen to it and be grateful for this experience, because it's showing you exactly where you need to go.**

I love myself
when I listen to my
regrets and work to
change my actions
for the better.

# 25 SELF-CARE TOOLS TO ENHANCE YOUR
# SELF-LOVE AND ADVOCATE FOR SELF-CARE PRACTICES

**1** **Create self-gratitude lists.** At the end of every day, say or write down three things that you are proud of yourself for. Making a self-gratitude list ensures that you celebrate yourself daily, are in the practice of feeling grateful, and are sending loving energy to YOU.

**2** **Sleep.** Make sure you set aside enough time to get a full night's sleep, whether that means going to bed earlier or allowing yourself a bit of a lie-in.

**3** **Exercise.** Moving your body is one of the best things you can do for yourself. Go for a run, for a bike ride, for a walk, head to the gym—whatever makes you feel good about your body and the care you're giving yourself.

**4** **Do some yoga.** This isn't just exercise or stretching. It's a way of moving and breathing that allows you to make space for yourself, to quiet your energy so you can hear your inner voice.

**5** **Dance.** You don't have to be Beyoncé to get your booty moving! Dance like there's nobody watching and set yourself free.

**6** **Eat well.** Start your day off right with a healthy breakfast, and make sure you don't skip lunch, either. Give your body the gift of healing, energizing foods.

**7** **Take your lunch break outside.** It's tempting to eat at your desk and work through lunch, but it's better for you—and for the work you do—if you take a break! If the weather's nice, eat outside under a tree, or at least take a quick spin around the block to clear your head.

**8** **Plan (and take!) a vacation.** We all need a break and some time away! It doesn't need to be expensive or a trip to the Swiss Alps or anything. Sometimes just a night or two in a hotel can do wonders.

**9** **Practice saying "no."** It gets easier with practice! If you're doing something because you feel you should, but you don't really want to, skip it!

**10** **Practice saying "yes."** Just as often, we don't allow ourselves to say yes to the things we really want! We feel obligated to stay home and make sure the kids do their homework, when really, we could say yes to ourselves and take a night off!

**11** **Spend time in nature.** Garden, hike, climb a tree, or just go for a walk, but get outside and get dirty!

**12** **Snuggle up to a furry friend.** If you have a pet, take them on a walk or hold them in your lap. If not, visit your local shelter and get in a little love time.

**13** **Get organized.** When your life feels out of control, put in some time for yourself to get everything straight in your head. Clean up your calendar, tidy up the clutter, and get rid of that overwhelm.

**14** **Do what you love.** Set aside some time for a hobby you enjoy, something that you're proud of.

**15** **Embrace that guilty pleasure.** There is no such thing! Pleasure is free of guilt, always. But do the thing you love just because you love it, no judgment!

**16** **Rearrange your furniture.** Sometimes the feeling of a new space can allow you to see new possibilities.

**17** **Explore and learn something new.** Try a new language or a new skill—challenge yourself!

**18** **Spend 5 minutes in meditation.** A little goes a long way, so there's no need to pull yourself into a pretzel and sit in silence for hours!

**19** **Call a friend.** Reach out to someone you haven't talked to in a while.

**20** **Donate.** This can mean donating money, working at a shelter, or volunteering as a tutor.

**21** **Give yourself a present.** Maybe it's a bouquet of flowers, a new pair of shoes, a cozy blanket, or a new yoga mat. You can also give yourself the simple present of spending time outdoors or just taking a break.

**22** **Light some scented candles or burn essential oils.** Aromatherapy *works*, girl. Certain scents can relax you, energize you, lift your spirits, and bring back joyful memories.

**23** **Dress up.** Looking good can help you feel good. Even if you're not planning on leaving the house, put on something that makes you feel gorgeous, just for you.

**24** **Wake up for the sunrise.** This one may not be so easy if mornings aren't your thing, but this quiet awakening of the day is a special gift you can give to yourself.

**25** **Write out a list of goals.** Dream big! Anything and everything is possible for you.

## Homework: Being a Self-care Goddess

Make a list of things that light you up. Let's call it a love self-care list. Include all the things you can think of. Write whatever comes to your mind without judgment or any limiting thoughts. After you're done, go through the list and mark down the last time you did that for yourself. Next, schedule these things into your days.

Then, call a friend and tell her about your newfound commitment to self-care and ask her to join you. Let her know that she is so worthy to have things in her life that light her up inside. Tell her what you love her and admire about her. Ask her in what ways she has been doing things for herself and in what ways she believes she hasn't been. Share with her what you learned about her sign and ask her how you can support her and hold her accountable for adding more self-love and care into her days. Support her with her list! Show her how to make self-care a priority, and set up a weekly meeting to support each other in this journey.

Imagine a world where women made self-care practices a top priority for themselves and joined together with their loved ones in supporting each other in having their practices be nonnegotiable. Imagine a world where we encouraged each other to dive into self-expression and do the things that fill us up and to have self-care on our calendars just as we would have eating breakfast, lunch, or dinner as a must-do during our days. We can do this! We can do this together. We can create a movement where

all women are taking care of themselves and creating space for each other to do the same. Self-care can become a part of everyday life, a part that you would never skip.

The way you take care of you reflects the amount of worthiness you have for yourself. Whether you realize it or not, you neglect yourself when you don't make self-care a priority. This can be conscious or unconscious. When you begin to treat yourself like the gift to this world that you are, you will not allow anything to take away your time for yourself. A goddess who knows her worth is dedicated to renewing and refreshing her body, mind, and soul because she knows how important she is. Take time to reflect on the following questions:

- Have I been taking care of myself?
- Do I realize the gift that I am?
- In what ways have I been neglecting myself?
- What do I need to change to show myself that I know how worthy I am?

> A woman who knows she is worthy celebrates and praises herself.

Let's show yourself and the world the incredible belief that you have in you. When you show the world your worthiness, you not only empower yourself, but you also empower others to do the same.

**Step 1: Trust**

The world is ruled by the happiness of women. How? Because when a woman is leading with her radiance, she can quite literally lift up the energy of any room and change the trajectory of the planet. When a woman is given the space to lead with her radiance, she trusts herself and she creates love and peace around her; everything she touches turns to gold. When a woman is judged and not given space to be herself, she is unhappy, she is unable to trust herself because of society's rules, and therefore the world suffers, and so does she. Her intuition and the power that she holds are blocked by the pressure of conforming. Pick three ways in which you will begin to honor your power by trusting yourself. For example:

- I trust myself when I have a sign that the situation is not right for me. I make the decision with my well-being at the top of my list.
- I will trust my intuition and do my best to not allow outside circumstances to force me to explain or trick me to be logical.
- I will lead with love and speak my truth in every situation.

**Step 2: Praise**

This step requires a partner. Grab your self-care sister or someone in your home and support each other in praise daily. The more you praise yourself internally and then show up for yourself by speaking the words out loud to someone else, the more your confidence will rise, and the more you will know that you love yourself.

Think of a partner, friend, or maybe a boss that has never complimented, acknowledged, or praised you. How does that feel? How does that show up in your performance or your connection to them? Do you feel appreciated, loved, and seen by people in your life that have a difficult time using words to acknowledge you? This is the same for how you praise and show acknowledgment to yourself. If you are not doing this, inside you feel the same way about yourself as those around you who do not show their appreciation. Pick three praises a day. Do this with a partner. Before we go to bed, my husband and I share our praises for ourselves. I also use these practices with friends in praise circles. Pull together a few friends or reach out to other girls in the GirlTalk community and start your own text thread! Every day you each send a message of praise for yourself and celebrate and encourage each other each time a woman is beautifully brave and bold in praising herself.

**Step 3: Pamper**

It is time that you start looking at pampering yourself as a necessity as part of honoring your mind, body, and soul. This can be done in various ways. It is up to you to discover the ways that work best for you. What are three ways that you will pamper yourself every week? See the list on pages 126 to 127.

**Higher Love Level:** Throughout your day, place your left hand on your right shoulder and caress it, this soothes you internally and lets your inner child know that you are there. It is an action, an affection that you can do anywhere to remind yourself that you are taken care of and looked out for. It is a very soothing and nurturing self-care and love hack!

# I KNOW WHO I AM

# Chapter 5

# FALLING IN LOVE WITH YOURSELF

**I AM WILDLY** in love with myself. Does that sound weird? Or egotistical? Maybe even delusional? It's not, I promise you. It's our natural state of being. Remember, we are naturally inclined to love. Think about it this way—do you love your siblings? Your friends? Your parents? Your partner or your children, if you have them? Whoever it is you care for, doesn't it feel *completely natural* that you should love them? Sure it does.

The part that can feel weird or hard is loving *ourselves.* But you know what? *That* is the crazy thing. The idea that it's weird to love yourself makes no sense at all. Love is unlimited, love is free, and deep down we know this and that is why we seek love in everything we do because we know it's unlimited, we know that it's free. To be the one to give that to yourself is one of the ways you can experience freedom. Some people will choose to say you have to define it, or that it's too hard, or that it's not possible. I believe that because you are on this journey, because you are here right now, that you won't be one of those people—at least not anymore, because you know deep in your soul that love is freedom. And with the practices of this book, you will begin to discover and deepen the unlimited love that is available inside of you. My favorite thing to hear is that it's easier said than done because then I would ask, "Are you not worth that?" Of course you are! You are worthy of freedom; you are meant for unlimited love, because that is really what you are.

You have compassion for the people you're closest to, right? Well, nobody is closer to you than you are! You spend all day every day with yourself. You are privy to your most secret thoughts and your wildest dreams. You know yourself better than anyone else ever could, and when you are disconnected from that knowing, it's because you got lost in all the BS around you, the stuff that isn't really you, the stuff that really isn't serving your highest self.

If you had a relationship like that with anyone else, you would care for them so much your heart would be spilling over with light and warmth for them. So why not you? What would it be like to love yourself even more than you love other people?

"Is it work to take care of yourself?" If you believe that it's work, then it's certainly going to feel like work. Saying that it's hard is not going to serve you. But what could feel hard is getting rid of the junk that has built up to keep you from loving yourself fully and freely.

**When you love yourself, you can love others even more than you currently do.**

Maybe sometimes that is what stops you, because love can feel scary. When you love someone, they can still annoy you. They can still mess up. But you love them in all their imperfections. And sometimes, you'll feel that burst of affection, that rush of heart-swelling warmth where you just look at them or think about them and you feel a glow, a sweet flood of tenderness. At that moment, you are happy solely because they exist.

It is possible to feel that burst of affection for yourself. And it is the most amazing feeling! *Nobody* walks around all day thinking, "Tra la la, I love myself so much!"

But the burst of an appreciation and deep feeling for yourself does happen each time you stand in your power and have your own back. I've felt it, and it's possible once you have the reference point to access it whenever you choose to.

I love myself when
I express who I am. Loving
me is knowing myself, it's
being the unlimited love
that I seek to find in others
and finding it where it has
always been, inside of me.

The first time I experienced this kind of self-love was at a moment when I was really struggling. Like so many people, I have a family member with addiction problems. It's been a challenge for all of us for years—half of my life, in fact. When he has spiraled, I have spiraled, falling into a lot of situational depression, neglecting myself to be there for him. If you have a loved one who struggles with addiction, this will all be incredibly familiar to you.

But this most recent time, I did something differently. Before dropping everything and jumping in to help him (which I knew perfectly well would only result in harming me and not actually helping him), I stopped for a moment. I asked myself, "What do I need to give myself in order to not go down that road again?"

I meditated. I spent some time alone. I spent some time with friends. I did all of that instead of immediately freaking out and jumping into a car to make sure he was okay.

I love him, and I want to help him, but I also love me, and I need to help myself, too. I detached from the situation, and *then* I stepped up to help. The situation still hurt me, but it didn't have as strong a hold over me because my first action was to take care of me. And here's the thing—because I was more sourced, meaning that I was more connected to myself before I came running to help, I saw that my family member came out of this situation better than he ever had before. It's addiction, after all, so I know that probably won't last, but it was still good to see. In that moment of taking care of myself first, I set an intention to come out of this situation being more in love with myself. And you know what? I actually felt those feelings. I experienced that heartwarming surge of affection *for myself.*

That moment served as a reference point. I knew that I was capable of experiencing that level of self-love, and if I had experienced it once, I could do so again.

And I have, since then. Again, not all the time at all hours of the day, but it happens more and more frequently and with more and more ease, even in times that would normally send me into a spiral of self-recrimination. For instance, not long ago, I was putting together a launch for my business. It was a huge launch, bigger than anything we'd done before . . . and, well, we blew it. My team and I had been working eleven-hour days for weeks, but something glitched, and the launch just didn't work. Thousands of people literally didn't receive our materials. I don't even know why. Was it Mercury Retrograde? Who knows?

This could so easily have sent me into despair and self-blame. After all, it's my company and this launch was my responsibility. But I resisted the impulse. I gave myself a moment to feel upset about it, but then I pivoted.

And I had a moment of just feeling really proud of myself. I *felt* it, the same way I would be proud of someone I loved for being strong and staying positive in the face of a challenge.

Being in love with yourself is something we should all be and the feeling of it is something that we should all experience. Everyone should have it, and I believe that everyone gets to experience it if they say yes to the commitment. Self-love is no different from wanting to experience romantic love, or to experience an adventure—it is something we all want and deserve. Writing *I love myself* on a sticky note is not the same as really feeling it. Falling in love with yourself is spiritual and soul-based. It is so much more than a confidence boost—it is a deep and profound love that will transform your life. How can you begin to love yourself in small ways? Some important steps you can take when learning to love and care for yourself are:

**STEP 1**  **Forgive yourself.** Be in the constant practice of forgiveness. Forgive anything that you may still be beating yourself up over. Know that guilt or regret (as we talked about earlier) isn't serving you anymore or anyone else, it's keeping you stuck in all those negative feelings.

**STEP 2**  **Pay attention.** Remember your promise to be unavailable for any mean girl behavior towards your own self? Pay attention to how you talk to and about yourself. Don't refer to yourself negatively. Say one positive thing about yourself every day when you look in the mirror. CHOOSE to look for the good. If you catch yourself putting yourself down, say three more positive things directly after you become aware that you are speaking negatively about yourself. For example, if you find yourself saying, "I can't believe this is happening to me again, it's all my fault or this isn't going to work out for you!" Stop, take a breath, and say to yourself, "Everything is always happening for me and always works out in my favor, this is not like last time, I trust myself."

If there are areas of your life you need help working through, try working with a therapist or counselor. It's okay to get help. We're not meant to do life alone. You are worthy.

**STEP 3** | **Practice repeating affirmations.** If you typically talk down to yourself, flip the script and turn your words into positive ones. Here are a few affirmations to try out:

> I love and trust myself.

> I am abundant and creative.

> I am worthy of love and attention.

> I choose to live in joy and love.

## LOVE YOURSELF, LOVE THE WORLD

**I TOLD YOU** at the very beginning of this book that if you are brave enough to love yourself, you will change the world, and the situation with my family member is just one example. I picked me for the very first time, and *that's* when I noticed an improvement in the situation. When you pick yourself, when you are proving to yourself that you love *you*, the universe will not only support you, it will support the other people in the situation as well. Maybe they will learn from your example and give themselves a little love and self-care. Maybe they will be forced to take care of themselves, because you're not immediately there to do it, and that will be the kick in the pants they needed. We never know how it will turn out, but choosing yourself is always for your highest good, and for the highest good of those around you.

I watched my family member's situation improve when I loved myself . . . and because addiction impacts everyone, that meant that the experience of everyone in my family improved. Because I took care of myself first, I was able to show up as the best version of myself, for them. Their lives improved because the person they love was showing more self-love, and they were able to breathe and have hope. And when they felt better, they improved the lives of everyone they encountered, from the grocery store clerk to their coworkers, and who knows how far it went from there?

> **Loving yourself has a ripple effect that travels farther than you can ever imagine.**

When you fall madly in love with yourself, you become in love with the world and everything around you. For the more joy and compassion we give to ourselves, the more we are helping others. Love is ever-expanding.

Falling in love with yourself is about being happy and living a peaceful life. When you're in love with yourself, you'll love your life and your experiences. You'll be happier. This happiness radiates outward energetically, so that it's not just your actions and experiences that improve the lives of those you come in contact with—there's so much more! Your positive energy lifts the general energy of the world, raising our shared frequency. As each one of us contributes to that positive energy, the frequency of the world will shift for the better, and the world as a whole will improve.

## LOVING YOURSELF IS AN ACT OF COURAGE

**WE SPEND A LOT** of our lives existing in survival mode, in a state of fear, and fear is what stops love from flowing. We are triggered by events outside of our control, by childhood wounds and traumas, and by the hurt other people cause us, inadvertently or not. We are afraid of the pain we might experience if we take a risk, or if we fail, or if we don't get what we want—and so we do nothing at all.

It is not possible to feel love in a state of survival. Fear is the opposite of love. Love is real and fear is not real; it is not the real you. Gandhi said that the real enemy is fear, not hate, and he would know! We think of Gandhi as this incredibly brave man who stood up for his people, but like all incredibly, beautifully brave people, he had his own fears to live with and walk through. He had failed at multiple careers, as both a lawyer and a teacher, and was afraid that he would never find a purpose in life. He was afraid of public speaking, and yet, in one of his first acts of protest, he spoke before a group of Indians in Pretoria that he had organized, urging them to join him.

He also had reason to know quite a lot about hate. At one point, he was confronted by an angry mob and severely beaten, but he refused to identify his assailants. He said, "They acted out of anger and ignorance, and if I do not forgive them, I will be as guilty of perpetuating hatred as they are." Time and time again he turned away from hatred, because he understood that hatred was rooted in fear. We only hate something because we fear it, and we know from Gandhi's writings that if you are led by fear, you cannot access love and compassion.

> **When you stand at a crossroads and need to make a choice, ask yourself whether your decision is based in fear or based in love.**

When I say based in love, I'm talking about what comes from your heart, from your highest being, from caring for the highest good and with no trace of fear. All decisions—whether as vast and impactful as Gandhi's path of nonviolence, or as simple as how to respond when someone cuts you off in traffic—are based in either fear or love.

When I made the decision to launch that new business venture, the one that backfired so spectacularly, I know now that I made the choice I did from a place of fear. I didn't know it at the time. I believed that I was looking at all the *good* it would do, at the huge difference it could make in people's lives, and for the difference it could make in the financial well-being of me and my family (which, like everyone, is something I have felt fear about sometimes). I focused on those factors, and I ignored my intuition. My soul was telling me that while this new project was definitely a good thing and absolutely for my highest good, and for the highest good of everyone that it would one day help, it was also a giant demand that I was placing on myself. The rushed timeline that I was putting on it meant that this project was going to drain me, and take me further away from my connection with myself, which in return could have a ripple effect on not just me but also those around me, those who look to me because that is how powerful each of us is. I would become so inundated with meeting the project's demands I couldn't be as present with my family, my friends, and myself. I knew, deep down, that I didn't have the time to do this project, plus show up fully for everything else I had going on *and* take care of myself, and that I was risking not only burnout but also my own well-being and the well-being of others.

In making this big business decision, I didn't listen to myself. I made my choice out of fear, rushed the timeline, and put myself and ultimately the project at risk. My decision did not come from a place of truly loving myself, of putting myself first, of choosing *me*. Even though I knew that it was the best decision for me and that it wasn't something I truly wanted right then, I was thinking about the external rewards and did it anyway, so it did not work out. In the end, it was an expensive lesson for me, but I will also never make that decision over myself again.

When you're faced with a choice like this, be brave. Be brave enough to not rush into it, to trust that what you are working toward will still be there for you when you're ready. Trust yourself and the universe to know that everything will work out. You can't mess up anything that is meant for you, so choose to be beautifully brave and not be scared of what will happen.

**Trust yourself because you love yourself so much.**

I love myself
when I trust my soul
to guide me in
my journey.

This is how you move from a place of survival to a place of true love and appreciation. It takes courage, but I have faith in you. Loving yourself might seem like it's taking a risk, but it's actually your true state of being and what you are meant for. It feels like a risk after years of being in a world that can feel scary at times, but it can also feel equally or even more so like complete joy, if you let it. If you let the years of becoming what you truly are slowly melt away by loving yourself, something amazing will happen—it will begin to feel like a scary risk to not love yourself and have your own back.

When you are in a state of fear, fear is all you can feel. You block out the feelings of love and any blessings that may be coming your way. Fear acts like a pair of blinders, allowing only negative things to come into view, keeping you in the cycle of fear. So, when you're in a state of fear, you are only attracting more scarcity, and therefore, more fear.

The antidote to fear is love. Now, you can't just flip off the blinders and *ta da!*— now you're in a state of pure bliss. Fear will grip you tight. But if you allow yourself to feel your fear, to bring awareness to what you're experiencing, your fear will relax its grip. It will let you move through it . . . and you can make your way back to love. It's a practice. It's an ongoing way of life. Your self-doubt, limiting beliefs, and all those other things that keep you in survival mode aren't just going to magically go away. They will always be there to some extent, because they're a part of what has made you who you are—and who you are is *wonderful.* Recognize that fears are there, get curious about those feelings, and then decide to make the down payment of faith on yourself and walk through to the other side.

Remember, bravery doesn't mean you're not afraid. Be scared, and then do the scary thing anyway.

## LOVING YOURSELF MEANS LOVING ALL OF YOU

**I KNOW THAT** for some of us, it can be easier to love ourselves at certain moments of our lives. Like when you've worked hard and achieved success and you're happy and you know that you're good at what you do, then sure! Self-love is a cinch! And that isn't really having love for self. That is just thinking because you achieved something you must respect and admire yourself now. It is doing to yourself exactly what you dread about others.

In society, we can get judged on our achievements or lack thereof, and when you only show yourself some praise and love when you "get it right," you are doing to yourself the exact thing that has you feeling small, or not good enough, or separate from others, to yourself. People get confused and think that when someone exudes confidence that means they love themselves. That is not a tell-all factor of self-love. Loving yourself is respect for who you are—it is a feeling, an unspoken commitment. It means being best friends with yourself and making decisions based on what is really best for you. The type of confident energy that comes from that is not the kind that screams to be heard in a room and is the biggest person in the room. It's the kind of confidence that doesn't scream; it just is. It is an unspoken energy, a love you cannot see that fills up the room with love, has others around you feeling love, feeling seen, and feeling included. It's the woman in the room who is laughing because she is in just so much joy. It's not the woman in the room who is laughing, carrying on, and screaming to be the center of attention while not allowing others to be seen. Somewhere along the line we got this whole confidence and self-love thing kind of messed up.

Everyone wants to be seen, and they will do anything to be understood. When we're feeling desperate or frustrated to be seen and understood, usually we cry out for attention or something outside of ourselves to heal that feeling. But in fact, your own soul is who wants to be seen by you.

> **Your soul is who wants to be understood by you, and you are who needs you to stand up for you.**

By seeing you, you break any need to be approved by others. By allowing yourself to see you fully and giving yourself compassion to understand where your needs come from, you then will not have anyone in your life who is toxic to your needs, who doesn't understand your needs or see you. So many times, desperation to make friendships or relationships work, or that constant story of going after the "wrong" person, being in the wrong relationships, is actually you looking to be seen in the wrong place—the place where you will never be seen. And if you stay there, you will endlessly be looking in the wrong place while your soul, your intuition, cries out. You may have just been looking to be seen in the wrong place, by the wrong person, until now.

So, what about when things are harder? What about loving yourself when you aren't a specific type of "success" yet, when you aren't happy, and when you are or have made choices that you aren't proud of? There are times when I would look back on my past self with judgment. I would be embarrassed, even ashamed.

The hardest times, the hardest parts of myself to love, are from my childhood. That might surprise you—after all, I was just a kid, right? But my childhood wounds are the source of a lot of my limiting beliefs, and so even though I can know intellectually that I was just a kid and deserving of love, that doesn't make it any easier to feel it. Again, *feeling* self-love means so much more than just saying, "Sure, I love myself."

When you find yourself slipping into a state of fear, it's often because you are remembering—consciously or unconsciously—something that happened to you when you were younger. We are shaped by our childhoods, by events both large and small, and our childhood wounds can stay with us. Our body remembers our life in a different way than our brains do, the parts we haven't yet healed are tucked away inside, and our inner child is always within us. Even if this is something you would rather look away from and pretend doesn't exist—*it does.* It's part of who you are, it's why you react in certain ways, it's why you feel a rush of fear, anxiety, or are flooded with emotion when certain triggers come up. It's why you hear of people "losing their shit" because you looked at them the wrong way.

I know I've definitely done it. Whenever things would be going well for me, whenever I was experiencing my dreams coming true, I would soon feel a negative emotion in my body. A lot of the time I would begin to self-sabotage. This was my body wanting to protect me. I wouldn't know what I was doing or why, I just kind of knew that I was feeling this negative, heavy sensation in my body whenever something amazing was happening.

It even happened on my wedding night! Isn't that supposed to be this perfect, dream event? Well, I sure didn't *feel* like it. We'd had the perfect day—imagine it, a wedding day that actually went perfectly! It was this glorious, fun celebration, an absolutely dream day. Josh and I went back to our room at the end of the night. He went to embrace me, and I remember getting this annoyed, heavy feeling. I'd just had the most amazing experience, and all I could think of was this overwhelming feeling of annoyance, like I was anticipating something awful I knew was about to go wrong. I had no idea where it had come from! It certainly had nothing to do with him—I knew I had just married the love of my life! So, what the heck was this?

I had already been doing a lot of self-work, but I hadn't done any work on my inner child. I'd gotten by for so long by keeping the faith and maintaining a positive attitude, but this experience forced me to go deeper. And I figured out that my childhood traumas were telling me that I always needed to be looking ahead for the next bad thing. If things were going well, then that meant they were about to get worse. And if something was amazing? Well, buckle up, because that meant I was about to get hit really hard. That feeling of heaviness was my body trying to protect me from some unwanted, painful surprise that my inner child thought was waiting just around the corner.

Looking back, I realize I was experiencing an "upper limit" problem. I had achieved such beautiful happiness in my romantic life, my business was growing, and my entire world felt like a dream. In this amazing moment, I had hit what I thought was my upper limit, that point where your ego tells you that you can't have more.

> **When we hit an upper limit like this, our ego tends to bring us back down below the line, back into our comfort zone.**

It does so by giving us negative thoughts or behaviors that could cause us to self-sabotage what we've achieved. Have you ever felt so happy, and suddenly found yourself imagining someone you loved passed away? Or perhaps you achieved a major career milestone, and in the midst of celebrating, began to wonder when you're going to lose it all? This is something we all face, but something we can all overcome. Now, whenever I feel myself hitting this point, I pause and ask myself, "How much love and happiness am I truly willing to have?"... And my answer is "Infinite!"

These things can happen at the craziest times. Triggers can come up when we don't expect them because everything has a much deeper association than it seems on the surface. If everyone chose to dedicate their life to loving themselves, the world would look like a much different place. Can you imagine a world where we aren't all so triggered all the time? People would respond from a whole place, not a wounded place. People would feel more empowered to speak their truth and have far fewer misunderstandings. When you are not aware of your triggers or not curious about them, you will respond to situations and operate in your everyday, from your triggers rather than from your heart. If you operate from your triggers instead of from your heart, you are not giving yourself love—instead you are functioning from a place of trauma and pain. This will in turn affect how much love you are giving and receiving, and essentially, affect the kind of life you want to live. If you respond from your heart, you are more likely to receive even more and come out of situations with the best possible outcome.

> **With all of your beautiful presence in this world you have the power within to heal those parts of you, clear anything that is in the way of that part of you that is *already beautiful*, and get yourself to a place where *you* can see the beauty, too.**

That means doing the work for your inner child and going back to those experiences, those painful moments that created your defense mechanisms and your fear, and giving yourself what you needed as a child at the time.

Let's imagine a woman. We'll call her Jessica. She's a novelist, and the mother of two rambunctious boys, she lives in a house with a giant yard where those boys can burn off some of their energy, and she loves her life every day. Yet she feels a sting of loneliness at times even though she is surrounded by everything you could have possibly ever dreamed of. What she doesn't love is looking back on her own childhood. It's not that it was so awful—her parents loved her, and she knew it—it's just not something she likes to think about.

She had been a lonely child. She was often caught up in her own imagination, lost in her inner world, so much so that the other kids thought she was weird. Maybe she *was* weird. And her parents noticed that she was on her own a lot and didn't have many friends, but they didn't really know what to do about it. Everyone just kind of went on with their lives. Jessica grew up, and eventually, by the time she got to college, she met other people who were caught up in their imaginations, and who were "weird" in the same way that she was. But it took a long time, and there were so many years that Jessica had spent alone. Even in her first year at college, she didn't know how to talk to people, or how to trust that they liked her. She didn't know how to be the kind of friend she wanted to be because she had never had a friend like that.

If Jessica were to look back to that time in her life, if she were to go back and love herself then, what would she need? What didn't she receive at the time? She had the love of her parents, but she didn't have their understanding or their help. She had her imagination, but she didn't have the love of friends, of people who liked her. In cultivating that love for herself, Jessica used her imagination. She thought about sitting down with her teenage self. She imagined re-parenting herself, with all that she knew now as a mother. She told her inner little girl that there were people out there who appreciated the creative person she had become, but that they were probably just as shy and lost as she was. She talked to her inner little girl as a friend, as someone to hang out with and tell secrets to. And as she imagined these conversations, she felt a surge of true, heartfelt love for the parts of her inside that needed someone to see her, to understand, to love her, and to show her compassion.

When we look back at the hard times, and at people who have hurt us, often in far more traumatic ways than Jessica experienced, we talk a lot about forgiveness. Forgiving the person who caused you harm is absolutely important . . . but it's not the whole story. You need to forgive yourself, too. We assign blame to ourselves just as much as we do to others, sometimes even more so, and finding compassion and forgiveness for ourselves is so important. It's showing yourself you are seen and forgiving yourself as easily as or easier than you forgive others. Forgiving yourself allows you to release the trauma you've been carrying and recognize that it no longer serves you.

Forgive yourself and show your inner child that it wasn't her fault. You won't really heal from your trauma unless you give yourself the love that you should have received at the time. Now, it might not always be so easy—and of course you should absolutely seek outside help in coping with trauma, whether that's therapy, counseling, or whatever else may work for you—but healing trauma starts with forgiving yourself. Shower that inner little girl with so much love. When you give love to a younger part of you, *all* parts of you will feel this pure self-love and complete compassion.

> Wake up every day and thank yourself for being the bold, beautiful, wonderful woman that you are.

## LOVE IN YOUR NATURAL STATE

**IF YOU'VE BEEN** unhappy or are having trouble feeling the love you want to have for yourself, it may be because you've lost sight of your natural self, the person you are underneath all the layers of limiting beliefs and societal expectations. All of these things that are put on us can lead us to lose sight of our purpose, of what we are meant to spend our lives doing. I got myself back on track by embracing my natural talents, by uncovering all that I had been told *not* to be, and embracing my loud, "too much" natural self!

But sometimes it can be hard to find our natural state, buried as it is in the rubble of other people's ideas about who we should be. I get this a lot from clients, actually—women who are successful, and whose lives from the outside appear great in every way, but underneath it all, they're miserable. I've worked out several processes to help them get back to who they are and were meant to be, to where they can feel joy in their lives and love for themselves as they live their purpose.

One of these involves going back to the beginning. We talked a lot in this chapter about childhood and how it can inform who you are today, but we mostly focused on the wounds that we can receive when we're young, and there's so much more there!

> **Childhood is the closest you can get to your natural state, and there are a lot of clues there about your purpose.**

When we're young, we're asked over and over again, "What do you want to be when you grow up?" Your answer then is your answer now.

Well, sort of. It's a little more complicated than that. If you wanted to be a ballet dancer when you were four, but now you're in your thirties and *Swan Lake* just isn't in the cards for you, you're probably thinking this isn't super helpful. A lot of us had childhood dreams that maybe weren't so "realistic", or at least looking back they seem that way but what you have to remember is that these are clues that can make you go, "Hmm, I wonder?" When you thought about being a ballet dancer, what was it you were longing for? Was it the beauty, the grace, the physicality, the movement?

Let's say it was the beauty. Your four-year-old self was swept away by the glorious costumes and the glamour. You could look at pictures of a ballerina and that would be enough. That tells me that it wasn't really only about dancing! You were lit up by the makeup and the clothes, so maybe something strong inside of you needs to have creativity in your life, you are meant to be expressing yourself in movement, beauty, and creation.

"I want to be a doctor when I grow up," is another common one, but it doesn't necessarily mean you need to head to medical school. What was it you admired about doctors? How did the idea of being a doctor make you feel? Was it really about getting in there with the blood, guts, and germs, or was it the idea of helping people? If you saw what doctors could do, then maybe what lights you up is supporting other people, helping them feel better and happier, and you don't need a medical degree to do that!

Or let's say you wanted to be an actress. If we unpack that, were you in it for the self-expression or for the acting? Whatever the answer, it doesn't *have* to mean Hollywood. Acting is about getting into another persona, and that can mean so many things. It can mean sales, being an attorney, being a novelist, or even being onstage. If your dream was about being self-expressive, then that just tells you that you need to be doing something creative and imaginative! Whether this is in your career or not, this is a telling point that these things and what they ignite inside of you is an important part of fully showing up for yourself.

Your natural talents can come through in your childhood ideas of what you wanted to be when you grew up, but they do require some translation. As a child, you went for the simplest, most obvious answer. You didn't really have the emotional intelligence and self-awareness to figure out what those answers meant. But you do now! So, take out your journal and list all the things you said you wanted to be over the years, and then break them down one by one. What was it you liked about being an astronaut or a firefighter or a veterinarian? How did the idea of being in that role make you feel, and how does it feel in your body now? It's the feeling you want to pursue, not the actual career! If you don't like what you do and you don't feel fulfilled, unbecome what isn't you and get back to what you *do* like and what *does* fulfill you.

There are so many answers in connecting to your inner child and going back to what you can remember or what you can connect to on a more spiritual level for the answers of what naturally lights you up and what your natural self is before anyone else told you who you are.

> **By exploring a more spiritual or connected side and showing yourself that you are curious about your inner child, you'll be able to find out more about who you are without all of the baggage that has been put on you through the years.**

Work this out on a piece of paper, get curious about yourself as a child, pay attention to movies, stories, or ideas that you feel a pull to, there's a lot of magic in there for you.

You can begin by:

**STEP 1**

Placing a picture of yourself when you were little on your bathroom mirror. Look at this picture and interact with it daily. She will come alive and you will both be able to support each other, heal, and get back to your power.

**STEP 2**

Write out what you wanted to be when you were younger, workshop what those things provided for humanity, what parts do you still resonate with? This isn't to say that you will go out and completely change whatever you are doing, but at the very least, you can add parts of you that you may have forgotten about into your life, whether it is through hobbies, activities, or maybe even a new side project.

**STEP 3**

Getting grounded in nature. To become very in tune with yourself you have to add nature into your practices. Anytime you feel anxiety, fear, or the feeling overwhelm you take yourself further away from your true nature or feelings and cannot fall in love with yourself. Go outside every day for at least 15 minutes. Touch the grass, the dirt, the sand. Walking outside can help reduce stress and pain. Set your bare feet on the earth to be instantly grounded. Give your worries away to Mother Nature, she will suck it up and take it away from you. A grounding practice like this will contribute to your overall all well-being and connectedness to self.

Astrology is also one of my favorite spiritual tools for figuring out what we really need. It can help you uncover your natural state, which will help you understand yourself. Astrology gives you a starting point. Of course, each of us is unique, and not every Leo will be exactly the same. A horoscope won't give you specifics, but it will help you figure out how to express the real, inner you that you love so much, and share her with the world. It can help you figure out what lights you up, what connects you to your true self, and what inspires you to do your best and most fulfilling work. You can use the link on page 205 to get more in tune with astrology if this is your preferred method of connecting with your natural state. I have created a system and process that helps you to connect to your sign and fall in love with yourself.

Are you ready to completely fall in love with yourself? The last process that I use is a twenty-one-day self-care experiment. You commit to twenty-one days of self-care practices. You will design these twenty-one days of rituals that bring you life, restore you, captivate you, help you relax, and invigorate you. You can start bringing self-care into your life as a nonnegotiable by saying "yes" to yourself and "no" to others. You can clear out your schedule for these self-care days and let people know that you have committed to a twenty-one day self-care experiment and you are not going to break this promise to yourself. You can use these self-care days to redesign your life, your practices, and begin to learn how to not only fall in love with yourself, but also learn what things you need to do that are special to your unique self.

While you are doing this self-care experiment you will also begin to add something daily into your life that will connect you to your deeper knowing. Take all the things you are learning throughout these chapters and customize what your self-care days will entail. Check out the resources page (page 205) for bonus material that you can use to dive in for some extra support and use to get guidance on mixing spirituality, grounding, astrology, and inner child work into your twenty-one-day experiment.

**To be in love with yourself is magic. When you love yourself fully, you radiate. Radiance is your birthright.**

# 15 WAYS TO DEEPEN THE LOVE INSIDE OF YOU

**1** **Practice self-compassion.** You know yourself more than anyone else and you deserve the kind of love that you would give to the person you love most, and that person is you.

**2** **Show up for yourself first before showing up for others.** Part of loving yourself is taking the time to take care of you first before running to tend to someone else. Sometimes, we forget about ourselves while we are busy trying to help someone else and not realize that we are causing more harm than good because we aren't showing up as our best selves. Take the time to take care of you first.

**3** **Forgive yourself.** We aren't perfect and there will always be things that we regret or feel guilty about. Not forgiving yourself doesn't serve anyone any good and doesn't allow you to move forward. We have to forgive ourselves in order to heal and let go of any pain or hurt in our lives.

**4** **Pay attention to how you talk about yourself.** Even if you are joking around, your mind, body, and soul can't tell the difference. Always speak highly about yourself.

**5** **Repeat affirmations.** Repetition goes a long way when it comes to affirmations. If you are constantly speaking good things to yourself, then you are feeding your mind, your body, your soul positive energy and you will be calling forth positive things into your life.

**6** **Fall deeply in love with yourself.** When you are in love with yourself, you fall in love with everything around you. You'll be happier and loving all of the little moments in life.

**7** **Make decisions based on love.** Ask yourself if you are making decisions from your heart and everything will start to fall into place.

**8** **Choose bravery over fear.** Loving yourself is an act of bravery and when you choose to love yourself, you are choosing to look past fear.

**9** **Love yourself all the time.** There will be times where loving yourself will be hard to do, especially when you are going through a tough time, but loving yourself means loving yourself at all times.

**10** **Be mindful of the "upper limit" belief.** We will hit those times when we think we don't deserve any more happiness because we think we can't go any higher or we believe that something will happen to sabotage our happiness. But love is infinite, and we can always have more of it. You are deserving of it all.

**11** Be aware and curious about your triggers. If you take the time to work on your triggers, you will be able to react to things from your heart instead of from a place of pain. You'll be able to see the clearer picture and give yourself and others love.

**12** Show up for your inner child. True healing happens when you give your inner child the love she needed at that time.

**13** Connect to your spiritual side. Grounding yourself in nature is a great way to connect to your spiritual side and has been known to have some positive effects on your body. By connecting to your spiritual side, you'll be able to explore who you really are without all the baggage that comes from the world. You'll experience love in its natural state.

**14** Have some fun with astrology. If you're having trouble figuring out what it is that you like to do or what will spark that fire inside of you, astrology is a fun way to explore the natural side of you. It may not be the most accurate for everyone, but you may find out some cool things about yourself by knowing more about your zodiac sign. Give it a try!

**15** Commit to a twenty-one-day self-care experiment. Design twenty-one days of rituals that restore you and bring out the best in you.

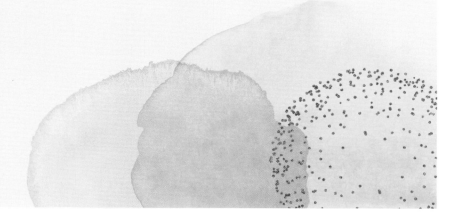

# Homework: Declare Your Destiny

Take your destiny into your own hands. The reward is an extreme sense of worthiness and love. Treating yourself like the goddess you are is not always easy. It does take effort, but every woman can design a deep love and life. You can decide your own version of what that looks like. Staying in relationship with yourself through self-care, self-expression, and positive habits creates a master of self-love. You become a master of declaring your destiny and loving self: you know what you need, and you give it to yourself. You know what you deserve, and you don't settle for less. You love yourself; therefore, you are aligned in all the areas of your life. To own your destiny, you must do more than spring-clean. You need to constantly be checking in on yourself and dedicated to an ongoing, attentive, and loving relationship with yourself.

This exercise can help you begin checking in on where you are. It can help clear your mind of all the things holding you back. You can do this alone, but it would be best to grab a partner, a fellow sister. When partnering up with a fellow sister you both will establish that there is a judgement-free, confidential zone, and that you are free to reveal whatever comes up during this process.

**Step 1:** You and your partner will each take a turn of 10 minutes asking each other questions for a couple of rounds until you are both satisfied that you have checked in on yourselves. I suggest doing two to three rounds of questioning. It is best to do it in person or virtually, as long as you can see each other, so that you can use eye contact and body language to hold space for each other while building up courage to speak your truths. Partner one will ask partner two questions that help partner two check in with herself, and then after 10 minutes, you will both switch, and partner two will ask partner one the same questions. The following are some example questions that you and your partner can take turns answering to help you and your partner get started:

**Round One:**

- How are you feeling right now?
- What are you needing more of?
- What is it that you really are desiring to have?
- Are you happy?
- What do you need right now to be happy?

**Round Two:**

- Is there anything that you need to clear and clean with someone in your life?
- Do you need support from me to hold space for you to do this?
- How can I support you?
- When will you do this?
- What are you declaring will change moving forward?
- How will you show up for yourself?

**Step 2:** Set a date in which you will commit to coming together again or doing this with yourself. This is important to do this check in at least monthly so that you can air out any feelings, vent, get clear, be supported, declare your desires, and create your destiny.

**Step 3:** Make a list of all the things you love about yourself that you have been told by someone isn't okay. Maybe it is that you are "too loud," "too happy," "too" anything. Free write and do not judge a single thought or things that come out. Make it a priority to continue to add to this list and review it every month.

**Higher Love Level:** Set a reminder on your phone with your favorite affirmation or something that is secret to you, that reminds you to speak your truth and check in with yourself, daily.

**If you are outgrowing things, expansion is happening. Let this be a reminder that you are right on schedule.**

# I WILL STAND BY ME

# Chapter 6

# NEVER LOSE
# YOURSELF AGAIN

**CHOOSING TO COMMIT** to whatever it takes to never lose myself again changed my life forever, and with that same choice you are about to make, this is about to happen to you too.

**THE IDEA OF** never losing yourself is about being there for yourself by standing in your power. You are a powerful being and you are someone who matters in this world. Everything you do has a ripple effect on the world around you, and that also means how you treat yourself and others impacts the world.

Oftentimes, we may think that our actions, our love, or our thoughts don't really matter, but that is where we go so off track. It all matters. We are connected to things bigger than ourselves. You may have heard people say, "Step into your power." You may have asked, or you could be asking now, "What does 'step into your power' mean?" Part of not losing yourself is more about standing in your power rather than stepping into it. Stepping into it suggests it's not something within you, it's something you have to step into, and that simply isn't true. Somewhere along the way you may have forgotten that. But don't worry, I am here to remind you that it's there, waiting for you to claim it and stand in it.

> **Your power is something that is always inside you. It's a part of you: it's your inner power, peace, and strength that you are meant to use to stand up for yourself and for others.**

So often when people feel lost or begin to discover what they want, they start showing up for themselves more, which is amazing! They often go down a path to find themselves and try different things out; they get on the bandwagon of "Yeah, that's right, self-love isn't selfish, delete, delete, delete," and they begin to throw up boundaries out of nowhere, cut people off at the drop of a dime (hello to the recent popular term *ghosting*, and the now widely popular "cancel culture" is a part of this behavior), and fall into this "I must be rid of 'toxic' people" mind-set, which is not so amazing. They begin to put their needs first by cutting out who they view as "toxic" people, using the idea that self-love isn't selfish as their excuse for doing this, not realizing that what they are doing is toxic in and of itself. This type of mind-set leaves room for more hurt, lingering unanswered questions, resentment, regret, and no chance for closure or peace. And while the person thinks they are "loving themselves" by doing this, they forget that we are all connected, so not only is there an impact energetically but also by running, ghosting, pretending nothing is wrong, or not addressing things at all, you are leaving a part of yourself unheard, misunderstood and not operating in a clean space. You could very well be missing out on an important healing moment for yourself and for someone else.

In your life you may have encountered avoidance in some way or another, perhaps you grew up in a "let's sweep this under the rug and not talk about it" type of environment, or you are in a friend group or relationship like that, you probably encountered avoidance in one form or another. Or maybe the only avoidance you experience is within yourself. Avoidance causes issues in your inner world whether you realize it or not, and it has a silent and slow power to get you out of alignment with yourself. On the furthest degree of the spectrum, you can lose or avoid yourself completely.

Trust me, I have done this during my own self-love journey, so I am not judging. In the work that I do and through the years of experience in these areas, I have truly learned that discernment, the ability to perceive well, is one of the greatest skills we can develop—that way you are able to observe instead of judge. When we observe, we can assess the situation better, take notice of things we otherwise would not have, and make a difference rather than judge and bring someone down. Avoidance is something I have experienced and supported thousands of women as they've worked through these issues. You are not alone. There was a time that I didn't know exactly how to go from avoiding my own needs to loving myself, having my own back, speaking my truth, and showing love to others at the same time. This was the case for me because, when I was growing up, we didn't talk things out and come to an understanding. Addressing things wasn't something I experienced. Many of my clients revealed to me they too were sent to their room when they were upset and not able to come out until they had calmed down. In any case, avoidance is a learned behavior from our environment that turns into a safety net.

For a long time, not knowing how to completely own who I was, speak my truth, and embrace uncomfortable experiences kept me in avoidance mode. I wanted to avoid confrontation so I could stay safe and be liked. Avoiding myself and my own voice for "courtesy" to others, or not wanting to "rock the boat," only ended up hurting one person the most: me. When you begin to make conscious choices to show up for yourself, you will begin to collect little reference points that will let you know what it feels like to completely be in love with you. These reference points will help you continue to make the choice to have your own back.

Choose you every time. You will learn something from each situation: You will learn who is okay with it and who is not. You will learn who is and who isn't meant to be on that journey with you. You will also learn who might need some lessons themselves and you can quietly send them love and send them on their way. But sometimes you might not want to know the truth because that means finding out who can handle being part of the journey with you and who can't. At the root of your intuition, you already know. Embrace the lessons that come with choosing you because you deserve to experience that wonderful feeling of inner love. No matter how amazing or how terrible things get, always fight for you. What have some of these lessons been for you?

Women can struggle with setting clear boundaries or knowing when they are setting one because they are hurt or hiding. This makes sense because of the pressure and standards placed on us. So how can you be sure that you are setting a boundary that is needed and not doing it out of fear? The next time you notice yourself feeling upset, taken advantage of or in a fight or flight, look at the prompts below and go through these questions to get clear.

Where in my life do I feel taken advantage of?

Where in my life have I caused this to happen and/or to keep happening?

What behavior do I need to change?

Does this person really mean to hurt me?

Is there something from the past that is triggering this situation?

What is it that I want moving forward?

Get clear on *your* standards. What are you available for and unavailable for? What type of relationships, friendships, experiences are you desiring and what is a "yes" for you and what is a "no"? Knowing these standards ensures that next time you find yourself in a situation in which a boundary seems to be broken or you are questioning that there needs to be a boundary placed, you can look to your standards. Similar to values, they are a compass for you in how you decide to live and what standards you place on your life. Let me share two of my standards with you to help you in creating or expanding on yours. One of my standards is in friendships, I surround myself with women who show up, clean up their energy, are committed to loving themselves, and committed to growth. This is my standard of who I surround myself with because I desire to have healthy friendships and trust in my relationships. If someone seems to be out of line from the standard you've created for yourself, check in with your standard, have a conversation with that person, and clear the air. If there is an issue and the space doesn't feel safe to clear, that is a sign for you to reevaluate your friendship, to be honest about it, and to create a standard of being available for supportive, sincere, and healthy friendships only.

A second standard of mine is within my marriage. Josh and I both share this standard, and we often and always take time to clean it up. We clear it up by addressing any issues, shifting anything that needs to be sorted out, cleaning up the energy, and clearing anything that needs to be voiced. Our standard is to always have each other's backs and not allow anything to come above our marriage. Many times, when we go off track, for example, putting work above each other or our well-being, we pause and begin to see where we need to put boundaries up, whether it's putting our phones away at a certain time or having a nonnegotiable weekly date night. If you need to reevaluate the standards of your relationships' quality, you will need to create certain boundaries in order to do so. The key is to be honest and clear about your boundaries with those involved, and not apologetic.

Getting clear on your boundaries is an art and a lesson. I am grateful for the lessons I learned while choosing myself over and over again. I am hopeful that you can find ways to be grateful for your lessons too, and from here on out, continue to choose to embrace the journey and all parts of it, including who you are and what you believe in. Because along your journey, there will be tiny lessons that will be calling you forth to help support you to get back on your way and deepen your love for yourself. These lessons make you a better partner, mentor, friend, wife, and human walking the planet. Because of these lessons, I am able to study others' negative behaviors and understand where they come from, without taking them personally. These lessons have equipped me in the work that I do that I love more than anything in the world. I get to share this with others so that we can all begin to fiercely love ourselves and lift others up higher than ever before.

After my own experience of not quite understanding how to navigate my self-love journey with bravery and grace, I noticed the same struggles or confusion often happened for other women. Recognizing this common pattern sent me on a mission to study behaviors, thoughts, and the world's understanding of self-love so that I could mentor other women who wanted to stand in their power and fully love themselves. I wanted to help these women who were not exactly sure how to navigate that. I watched many women, some of them friends, others who are clients, who have very strong boundaries, are blunt, and are what they call "unapologetic." They can cut someone off at the drop of a pin because that person did something they didn't like, yet they still fear losing people. It makes sense that they would fear losing relationships because they were operating under an unspoken inner rule that they made up and were unconsciously removing people from their lives whenever someone did something they didn't like or that hurt them. At some point, the words *toxic* and *boundaries* became very popular catchphrases. But there aren't toxic people, there are only toxic relationships.

# "TOXIC PEOPLE" AND TAKING RESPONSIBILITY FOR YOUR PART

**THERE ARE TWO** types of toxic relationships: ones where the person feels like an energy sucker and a narcissist, who continues to hurt you and others to a degree that it is not safe to be around them. And then there are the situations and relationships that are simply not in alignment with your vision for yourself, with the standards that you are setting for your life and with what you need in order to fully love yourself and be committed to the relationship with yourself for the rest of your life.

I had an experience with the latter type years ago. I was in a friend group that I loved for a while, a sisterhood for that time in my life. Having "girl time" has always been very important to me. I look back on these friendships and appreciate so much and have some amazing memories. But, at some point, there appeared a tiny voice inside of me telling me that I wanted to do different things, talk about different topics, and connect with my friends on a deeper level. I didn't always care to talk about fashion or relationship problems, and I was so tired of gossiping and avoiding tough conversations with friends. This little voice was always with me, but I didn't really know what to do about it or where to find what I was looking for.

As I began to become more committed to my own happiness and alignment, I got deeper and deeper into loving myself. I thought I could do this and share what I was learning with my friend group. I didn't want to lose them, but because we were interested in different things, we were growing apart. That voice inside kept getting stronger and stronger, but I didn't have guidance on what to do. I hadn't met anyone who wanted the same things as I did in a friendship. More and more, I was craving a level up in all parts of my life.

As I grew, I felt further from them, but I still kept holding on. I would go to our weekly dinners and barely speak because I couldn't relate to the conversation, and I felt that if I said what I was going through or what I thought I would just be talked about behind my back. And while I stayed miserable trying to make something fit, I felt even more lost because I stayed quiet and tried to drown out that voice inside of me. I slowly told my inner self that my feelings didn't matter. While I may have been growing in my desires, I was silencing the part of me that wanted to be free because I didn't want to be alone. Finally, I realized that being in a group where I couldn't be myself without being talked about or causing a fight meant that I was already alone. I was not only abandoning myself but was also preventing myself from having the freedom to expand and the chance to meet some amazing people who might understand and accept me. Part of me thought those people didn't exist.

I wasn't equipped with the tools to talk about what I was experiencing, and I realize now I wasn't exactly clear on what was going on with me either, so I began meek attempts to express how I was feeling. I led with what I thought they were doing wrong, but the conversations would never amount to anything other than more gossip and misunderstandings. All sides kept trying to ignore the problems in the group, and each person kept going on pretending everything was okay but still feeling hurt. Finally, I was invited on a trip with them, and even though I knew I shouldn't go, I wanted to make one last attempt to get our friendship back. As I was making plans to rearrange my schedule and make the trip work (while slowly abandoning myself and not being honest with myself or them), I found out that the trip had not only been planned and booked, but it was also happening at another time than when I was told. All of the time and work I spent to move my schedule and bend over backward to fit into something my soul didn't even really want backfired. Even though at the time I thought I was so hurt by these women, what I was really hurt by the most was that I had been ignoring myself and my own feelings.

Later I realized that to them it must have felt like I had cut them off out of nowhere even though I had been feeling removed from the group for a while. I stopped answering their calls, I didn't address the things I heard they were saying about me behind my back, and I avoided their texts or followed up with short responses. As I am writing this, I still cannot believe how I handled the end of our friendship the way I did. But I hadn't learned how to stand in my power, call others forth, and speak my truth yet. And yes, I mean calling others *forth*, not *out*. Calling others forth is a practice; calling people out is wanting to do exactly that. You call them out, and then what? You get an award for embarrassing someone and proving your point?

> **The intention must be to call them forth, take a stand for them while holding your truth, share what you experienced, and give them a chance to change.**

A way to call someone forth is to not blame but to be clear and take responsibility for your experience. For example, "When you did (specific action) my experience of that was (share what you experienced)". When they don't take the chance, you hear the message loud and clear and move forward.

Years later, I cannot remember exactly when, I apologized to them. And though I never received an apology from them, I was okay with that because I had learned that in order to not lose yourself you must stand in your power, speak your truth, take responsibility for your part in the situation, and release any toxicity that you are holding on to. I was holding on to negative energy by not clearing things with them and being honest about what I wanted and why. I have very little idea what is going on in their lives now, but what I do know is that I still have love for them. I wish them the best, and I am completely cleared and free of my behavior, whether warranted or not, because I loved myself and them enough to turn the mirror around and take a hard look in it. I took responsibility for what part was mine. I hold no grudges, and if I saw them, I would run up and give them a big hug (if they'd let me!). It is important to take responsibility for your actions, because only then are you able to release resentment or any negative energy within yourself. You do it for you and many times you begin to heal two people in the process.

# TAKING RESPONSIBILITY FOR YOUR ACTIONS SO YOU CAN HEAL

**TAKING RESPONSIBILITY FOR** a relationship gone wrong is a huge part of personal development and inner growth. Sometimes we are so quick to judge the other person for the part they played in a relationship that we forget to look at ourselves and the role we played. We like to have a villain in the story and blame everything on the other person because it's harder to take a deep dive into ourselves and do the inner work to figure out what we can do to love ourselves and others more. Now, I am not saying that you have to keep "toxic" relationships or keep in contact with anyone or anything that contributes to "toxicity" into your life. It is completely okay to let go of what is not serving you, and that includes people. What I am saying is that there are times when we need to look at the relationship from a whole different perspective so that we can understand what we do or don't allow in our lives. For instance, if you keep going back to that same partner who keeps cheating on you, at some point, you have to recognize that something inside of you is saying that this is what you're worth—that this is the kind of love you are accepting.

> **Taking responsibility for your role allows you the space to heal and grow.**

There may be things that you are doing, like not communicating how you feel in the moment, that is harming the relationship. The other person has no way of knowing how you feel unless you reveal that to them. So, if you don't communicate and the person keeps doing something you don't like, then that doesn't necessarily mean they are "toxic." But it does mean that you are allowing them to treat you badly or cross a boundary that you are not okay with. In the end, you are hurting yourself by not telling the person what you are not comfortable with and you are not allowing yourself room to heal from the hurt this person is causing you. By telling them what is going on, you are also giving them the opportunity to fix it so you can move forward in love, whether that is by making the relationship healthier or by letting them go and moving on. We need to realize that we have a role to play in what we allow to enter and continue to be in our lives. Here are some steps to get you started in taking responsibility for your inner healing.

**STEP 1**

**Know yourself, your triggers, and where they come from.** Our triggers are reminders from our past painful experiences. At some point after being hurt, we begin to develop defense mechanisms that we are not always aware of and we then develop a default response to certain circumstances. This default response is linked to past traumas or wounds, and when something happens to trigger (no pun intended) this response, we react with old patterns.

Start to become aware of your triggers by taking notice of the emotions as they come up. Noticing these emotions is incredibly empowering and useful for healing and living a free life that feels lighter. Most of our responses in situations and our perceived perspectives of what is being said or done are influenced by our triggers. When you start to become aware of your triggers, you can begin taking responsibility for the way you respond to things. Taking responsibility leads to healing because you feel a sense of understanding. Triggers can bring up emotions or feelings—fear, jealousy, anger, or loneliness—that do not belong among other feelings. One way to get familiar with your common triggers and what is behind them is to journal about them and inquire about the situations that trigger you. You can do this is by writing down the experience, then asking yourself what was triggering about it, next to the experience.

How did this experience or event make you feel?

What did it feel like in your body?

What message did you tell yourself about it?

Where can you heal in this?

As you continue to do this every time you feel triggered, you'll not only gradually begin to become very aware of your triggers and where they come from, you'll also be able to shift quicker, take on a new meaning in the situation that will serve you and you will begin to notice when triggers come up in the moment and intervene before they consume you.

**STEP 2**

**Give others grace and choose to believe in the best of humanity.** When we were born, we were not born critics. We were open and curious. There is a reason that the phrase "hurt people, hurt people" came to be. As you love yourself more, and the deeper you stand in a power that is love, you find compassion for yourself and also for others. It doesn't mean you have to like everyone, be around people you do not feel safe with, or not speak your truth.

In fact, you do this even more because you are so at home with yourself that you know it has to be said for your greater good and for others. This means you accept the gift to send love to others no matter what, to give the benefit of the doubt, and be open and curious about things before you judge, label, or decide what it is. When we judge, label, or make decisions before knowing we are making choices based in fear, we are in our triggers and can miss a big opportunity for ourselves and others. We miss out on things like connecting even deeper with that person, learning more about yourself, or missing out on some magic that might be hidden there, and because you are choosing not to be open, it will pass you by. You will lose nothing by first allowing the benefit of the doubt. This will stop paranoia, allow truth to flow in, and open you up to new possibilities, perspectives, and opportunities. When we are open to what's true, we can manifest the best possible outcome for ourselves and others.

**STEP 3**

**Do not put others on a pedestal.** When we put others above us, we diminish ourselves and we set ourselves up with our own unkind standard that we will never meet because it's not a standard that is meant to be met. Putting someone else above or making them better than you is silencing yourself. You will never feel good enough when you put someone else's beauty, talents, achievements, or anything above your own and make them better than you. This is the same with putting people we love on a pedestal, for when we place them above us, we set them up to fall. Because no one is better than any other person, when we put all our expectations and desires into someone, we build them up to be more than human and we leave no room for mistakes. Inevitably, there will be misunderstandings and people will make mistakes, so if we place someone on the shelf of perfection, once they do something we view as a mistake, they will fall from our pedestal and our disappointment will rise. When you are able to know yourself and have compassion for yourself, you are able to do the same for others. You can only give or do for others at the capacity that you give and do for yourself.

We are all similar yet so different, and we all make a difference in our own unique ways. Society has created this flawed system of "better than," and in turn, there are a lot of pedestals being built and a lot of disappointment and judgment because of it.

**STEP 4** — **Declare what you have learned from the situation and what you will do differently moving forward.** Make it a practice to ask yourself what you contributed to the situation. Do this so that you only take responsibility for your part and not more. We have learned as women to over apologize. Taking responsibility is loving yourself because you are able to stand in your power and speak for the part you played and nothing more. You'll also know that you did play a part so that you can acknowledge it, release that energy, and learn from it for next time. Loving yourself is choosing to do what's best for you, and what's best for you in situations of conflict is to learn, clear the lower vibration energy, and move forward. Remember that everything is energy and if there are emotions that are left behind and not cleared up, you will have little energy blocks that build up and lead to bigger issues.

Now, you may be wondering about people who truly are toxic for you, the people for whom no matter what you do and say it won't ever be enough. You cannot have them both in your life and fully be loving yourself. This is one of the many reasons why it's vital to know yourself and take care of you, because it will become easier and faster to spot them, send them love, and send them on their way. You will love yourself so much and know yourself so well that you will understand they are not for you. Taking a stand for someone means loving them, even if they don't like what you have to say.

> **Taking a stand for yourself means speaking your truth and trusting yourself, even when that means you are going to possibly lose something or someone because of it.**

If you lose that person because you spoke your truth, you were going to eventually lose them anyway. So, choose yourself; show yourself that you trust yourself and will show up when you are needed. In order to stand for others, you must first stand for yourself. You must decide to love yourself so hard and so big that you can then inspire those around you.

When you speak your truth, take responsibility and let go of the need to be right, prove something, or avoid conflict. You will then feel comfortable navigating and experiencing your feelings, working through things, learning, growing, and beginning to vibrate at your highest radiance. As you stand in your power and allow yourself to vibrate as your most radiant self, you will see your life being surrounded by more and more people who lead and live the same way.

If you choose to ignore yourself, you will only keep attracting people who aren't in alignment with your highest self. You will continue to come across or be in relationships with the "wrong" people, whether it's a business partner, romantic relationship, or friendship. When this happens, you will feel alone, disconnected, and out of alignment. There is a lesson that needs to be learned here if you keep coming up against this. Until you decide to learn the lesson and do something different, you will continue to manifest the same type of people in your life and repeat the same patterns until you begin to listen to your inner knowing and complete the lesson that was meant for you.

Some people struggle their entire life with this lesson, continuing to attract the same type of problems, issues, or people and not understanding why. Maybe you have been there before; maybe you are there now. Is there something that keeps repeating itself that you deep down know isn't right for you? Or do you feel something that might not necessarily be so terrible, but it feels heavy or like something you have outgrown? Or is it simply becoming clear that you don't want to experience the same things anymore?

If yes, why do you think you are holding on to it? If not, take an inventory of all the areas of your life and check in with yourself. You deserve to be in constant connection and communication with yourself so that you continue to walk the path that your soul is meant for and not get lost along the way.

**When you hold on to things that are not meant for you anymore it's like drinking a tiny poison and slowly just letting it eat you up from the inside out.**

# GIVING YOUR
# FEELINGS A VOICE

**TO SHOW UP** for yourself, you must give your feelings a voice. When you ignore them because you're scared to lose someone or something, you lose yourself instead. When you give your feelings a voice, you begin to empower yourself to live in more freedom. You begin to understand your feelings in a very real and life-altering way. You begin to see where these feelings may be coming from and why, and you are able to clear that stuck energy in your body weighing you down. Each time you ignore a feeling, think of it as an energy of the frequency of that feeling and how that can build up over time. Your body keeping score is not just about trauma, it's also about the trapped emotions that have not been cleared or let free.

Our feelings can be buried by years of not expressing them, years of doing "the right thing" or not saying anything because "if you don't have anything nice to say, then don't say anything at all." This confuses you into thinking that if what you're feeling and your opinions are not "nice," then you should not share them. I'm not talking about kindness here, I am talking about giving your feelings a safe place to be free and abandoning the world's expectations of you. So, decide right now: what is more important to you, the opinions of others or your own physical, mental, and overall well-being? Without well-being, what do you have? You need to practice and care about yourself and your own well-being so that you can walk through fear, rise above difficulties, and experience what you desire in your life. Your well-being should be at the top of your list, and this requires loving yourself and prioritizing the relationship with yourself.

You've probably heard the expression "clear the air." Think of giving your feelings a voice in terms of clearing the energy. If you are keeping your feelings inside and expecting to be fully alive, you will wake up one day and wonder why you are so overwhelmed, stuck, or bored. This has happened to me more than once as well as any client or most any woman I know, and what I always find is that somewhere in my life and theirs we were not sharing our truths and not giving our own feelings a voice. You must first begin to create safe spaces to express your feelings and doubts; otherwise, they will fill you with resentment and unexpressed emotion.

Have you ever said, "Oh, it's okay, no big deal" or "I'm just not going to give that any energy"? Meanwhile, inside you feel like something is unresolved? That's because sometimes there is a tiny step missing and everything really doesn't feel okay at that moment. Do what you have to do to release and resolve any issue so you are able to move on with clarity and clear the energy.

We must not only learn to express ourselves but also let go of what is not meant for us, such as being a "good girl" and holding on to everything until we burst or until we hold it like poison inside and wake up wondering why life isn't what we thought it would be. We must find a safe place to clear, to get the energy *out*. This will look different for everyone, but here are some of my favorite ways to clear any residual energy:

**Screaming** into a pillow is a great energy release when you feel frustrated, stuck, or angry.

**Dancing** ignites joy, gets energy flowing, and releases energy not serving you! The more free these moves are for your body therapy the better, no choreography needed here.

**Shaking** works great to release tension in your body (take the term "shake it off" literally!).

**Tapping** against something, particularly with your fingertips on specific meridian points, while talking through traumatic memories and a wide range of emotions, helps you focus on the issue that you wish to figure out.

**Breathwork** is a great way for you to ground yourself and relax.

**Healthy venting** is a healthier way of speaking out your frustrations. Say bye-bye to gossip and telling ten people the same story over and over, and adding more hurt into your body, there is a new way!

Notice I say "healthy venting." This means giving yourself a safe place to say what you need, no matter how illogical or irrational, so that you can release the energy. You might even hear yourself say it and realize that it's not true or it's not as bad as your mind had you believe. Finding a healthy way to release the negative energy increases your well-being.

Other safe ways to let go of negative thoughts is through a trusted mentor or a friend that you can vent to without judgment. Or you can do a complete journal dump and then throw out the paper afterward. Venting only goes wrong for people who want to hold on to the issue and have no plan to release it and move forward. Then it could become a habit, an addiction, or a negative mind-set. That is not you, though. You are a powerful force, here to be different, to live an extraordinary life in love with yourself.

So, one of the most powerful things you can do for yourself is to begin to express yourself and turn that expression into your power. When you need to give your feelings a voice privately, vent it to a trusted person and in a way that you have designed for yourself. Remember, releasing this energy is vital for your inner and outer health, because what is going on inside shows up on the outside, whether through visible manifestations or through the hurt you place on others and yourself.

**Part of healing is acknowledging your feelings and giving yourself a safe place to talk about them.**

When you stand into your power, you will become unapologetic about who you are and what you need. You will set standards for yourself and make decisions for your life and what *you* want it to be. You will pay attention to the emotions that come up and listen to your intuition rather than the opinions of others.

What will it look like to truly love yourself and give yourself that unlimited power? You'll wake up excited to spend time with *you*, happy to be in your body, to look and feel great. You'll be excited to move your body, whether it's exercising, dancing, or making love. You'll look forward to the work you want to do in the world and enjoy surrounding yourself with people who lift you up. You will be fully yourself in every expression you want to be. You'll speak your truth loudly, living your life as all that you are.

**You deserve to be your number one fan, because when you love yourself you possess something that is unlimited, and that is the ultimate freedom.**

I love myself
when I give a voice
to my feelings and
speak my truth.

# HOW TO BE HONEST WITH THE PEOPLE IN YOUR LIFE

**ALWAYS CHOOSE TO** speak your truth and give yourself the permission you need in any situation, including the permission to take a minute if you need to. When you make these choices, you are showing the universe that you believe in abundance. When you stand in your power and always believe that things will work out for you in the end, you won't be scared to lose anything or anyone, and being honest with the people in your life will be a nonnegotiable for you. Here is how to begin being honest with your loved ones.

**STEP 1**

**Be honest with yourself first.** Access how you feel about the situation or the experience that is happening or has happened. Get radically honest with yourself about what comes up for you in certain situations and what you are and are not available for. When you know the answer, building the beautifully brave muscle of always sharing in honesty becomes much easier.

**STEP 2**

**Set an intention.** Set intentions for sharing and creating honest relationships with yourself and others. These intentions will serve you for cocreating with the universe the kind of energy and experiences you want to manifest in your life.

**STEP 3**

**Remember that honesty is love.** Being honest with yourself and others is the way that you stand in your power and give unconditional love. Love isn't not telling the truth (even when it doesn't feel that way); it's taking a stand for truth and love no matter what the circumstances are. Taking a stand for yourself to speak your truth is an act of love so strong its empowerment feels like electricity. Taking a stand also means loving yourself because you are choosing love over being liked. In society, we have learned to sweep unpleasant things under the rug or not rock the boat, but when you aren't being honest with yourself or others, you hold them back and you hold yourself back as well.

# HOW TO HAVE HARD CONVERSATIONS

**CONFLICT IS INEVITABLE.** What matters is how we have conversations and that we have them. This could be the difference between drifting apart or becoming closer. But you won't have your own mental health and energy sucked away because of something you aren't releasing. You deserve to have that peace for yourself and for your energy. Here's how to start having important and difficult conversations.

**STEP 1**
**Speak from the first person.** Use language like "I feel" or "I need," instead of "You did this" or "You're not."

**STEP 2**
**Own the story you created about this conflict.** "When X happened, I made it mean . . ." or "The story I am telling myself is that . . ."

**STEP 3**
**Release any judgment and practice leading with love.** Instead of saying, "Why can't you . . ." say, "Can you help me understand this more?"

**STEP 4**
**Mirror the other person.** Repeat back what was said to the person you are having a tough conversation with so that they can hear how you are interpreting what was said to you. Try saying, "What I hear you say is XYZ" or "Am I hearing that right?" This way, they have a chance to clear up a misunderstanding and they know they are being heard.

## CREATE A SAFE PLACE FOR YOURSELF AND OTHERS

**THINK ABOUT HOLDING** a safe space for someone you love to share their feelings and what they are going through. How does that make them feel when you do this? It allows them to open up, be seen and heard, and either move through what they are experiencing or embrace it more. Now as much as people need to have this grace from other people, they need this even more and more often for themselves. You can feel when it is safe to express your feelings. You know when you are pushing your true feelings down, ignoring them, or not paying attention to them. People can often tell whether you are being honest with them or not (though they might not follow through with their initial feeling), just like you know when you aren't being honest with yourself.

> **Therefore, it's important to create a safe place for yourself to express your truth.**

To create a safe space at home, find a corner or an area that you can retreat to that feels comfortable to you. This could look like placing a few fluffy pillows on the floor, lighting a candle or diffuser, and dimming the lights. This could also be created outside, in an environment that you find peaceful. When times get stressful, know that you can always come back here as a form of retreat, relaxation, and reflection. Your safe space quite literally can be an actual place and it also gets to be inside yourself. You can create a safe space inside of yourself by being more self-aware, saying more kind words to yourself, getting clear on your truth, facing your fears, giving your voice power, and feeling your undivided attention so that they feel safe inside you to show themselves clearer. Once your soul and body can feel that you will be there, you will listen, you will feel safe and secure inside yourself.

## PLEASING EVERYONE BUT YOURSELF

**ARE YOU A RECOVERING** people-pleaser? Or perhaps a people-pleaser to the core? Is it something you have been working through? We all have moments like this in life where we feel we have to please everyone but ourselves.

In 2010, while I was living in Nashville, I had this dream inside me that was building, but my actions and what I was focused on weren't matching up to the dream. I had moved to be closer to my family again and thought that was what I needed, yet when I got back there, I still felt what I would describe then as a lost feeling. The way I describe it now is a feeling of unalignment. I wasn't quite sure what to do with it or what it was telling me. I had been listening to everyone else's advice and hearing their thoughts on my life through their own lens. I imagine you have gone through a similar situation where you felt like you had to please others so they could be "proud" of you or where you feel as if you were behind in this race we call life.

I was surrounded by people who were getting married and having kids, and I had never even felt like I had loved anyone. At my friend's wedding, I remember crying, feeling so out of place, and wondering, will I ever do this? Do I even want this? What's wrong with me? I hadn't fully lived yet, and I had a big dream that I wasn't quite sure how to follow. My family had spent so much money on my education, and I was working to be able to get my master's degree, something I thought I was supposed to be doing, something that would bring me peace and purpose, yet it wasn't aligning, and I felt like a failure.

One of my best friends from college, Brittney, called me. She was going to Australia with a group of women and insisted that I fly to meet her in Los Angeles and join them. But it made me feel even worse because I felt like, once again, everyone had their life together and how in the world was I going to figure out how to afford this luxury trip to Australia? But she insisted that I go, and before I knew it, she had already booked the trip for me and wasn't taking no for an answer.

I was so grateful and excited. Her act of kindness meant the world to me, and at a time where I was feeling so lost it gave me some hope. I felt like someone believed in me because of this simple invitation. I had only been out of the country one other time, when I lived in Italy and traveled to Paris and London, and it was my most amazing life experience to date. I felt that same excitement and wonder as I boarded my flight to meet them in LA. We were flying business class, and I was secretly freaking out because I had never flown business class before. While I was both excited and completely in comparison mode, I decided that I would be grateful for the opportunity and stop worrying, at least for the rest of the trip; I could get back to worrying when I got home.

We arrived in Sydney on New Year's Eve, and we rushed to our hotel to get changed. The women had arranged for us to ring in the New Year at a party on a barge in the middle of the harbor. As we watched the fireworks over the water, I realized two things: I had been living my recent days pleasing others and worrying due to my pleasing of everyone else but myself. I looked out over the stunning views of the Sydney Harbor Bridge and somehow realized that I could start to believe in my big dreams again. Ringing in the New Year in Sydney opened me up to other possibilities, to possibilities I had believed in when I was a child.

I learned a really valuable lesson that night. I learned that the more I worried, the more I told myself I didn't believe in my own capabilities. I didn't want to do that to myself anymore. I didn't exactly know where I was going to start or what my next step would be, I just knew that I had made a decision to do something different and that I wanted to take care of myself. If you remember when we started this journey together in the introduction, I mentioned that in 2011 I picked up and left all my plans behind and moved to Los Angeles. This trip was the beginning of that beautifully brave move.

The lesson here is to remember that you need to spend less time pleasing others and more time pleasing yourself. You can't live a happy and fulfilled life if you spend it trying to please other people, because, like me, you will find yourself feeling as if you have failed in life, and you won't know how to move toward your bravery. There will be moments where you feel like everyone else is doing something that you are not, and you'll fall into the comparison trap we discussed earlier. I'm here to tell you that you are enough—always remember that. Your time will come. You are running your own race. And if you are feeling stuck because you are worried about what people think of you, spend some time giving yourself love and kindness. Think about what you want to do. Take that small step to your big dream today.

It's easy to feel as if you have to do something because someone else is doing it or because it will make someone feel happy for you, but your life is *yours*. Only you will have to live with the decisions and choices that you make, so take a risk toward your happiness. Live the life you want and don't spend any more time pleasing others. You will never win by pleasing other people because nothing will ever be enough, and you will never find that thing that makes you spark. It is human nature to search for our purpose in life, and if you don't find that for yourself, you will never be satisfied. You will always feel lost— like you are searching for something, like part of you is missing. By switching the focus back to you and your needs, you allow yourself the opportunity to discover and explore the things you enjoy doing.

**Focus on yourself and do that thing that makes you light up on the inside.**

For me, it was a simple invitation to an incredible trip that led me to take a step back and look at the beauty of my dreams. For you, it can be something as simple as saying "yes" to that thing you really are afraid to say yes to.

# DISCOVER YOURSELF AGAIN

**DURING THIS SELF-LOVE** journey, you will rediscover yourself. In the process of loving who you are, you will find out exactly what you need in order to give yourself the best love of your life. It will take some time to discover yourself again and to smash the self-love myths that have surrounded you your whole life. But once you get there, you will never go backwards to where you were, you will only grow and move forward because you have a different reference point and knowledge.

> **It can take someone years to realize that they are not living a loving life or to make a change, so no matter where you are in life, it is never too late to discover who you are and embrace that person.**

Take the time to explore things that ignite the fire inside. Go on that trip, say "yes" to that interview, take that new promotion, start that new business, get that new degree. Start a relationship with yourself and learn what your likes and dislikes are. Let go of things that are taking you away from your true self even if it's the scariest thing you have ever done.

On my trip around Australia, I realized that the other women on the trip were also there to find their way back to themselves. One of the women, Farah, had decided to get away because she was at a point where she had not experienced her own life. She was raised in a culture where women didn't have a voice: everything was decided for her and she was completely miserable. She explained how she felt trapped and sad. She struggled because while she financially had everything she could possibly ever need, she really didn't know herself because she was never allowed to express her true self. She stayed longer on the trip, spending time exploring the woman she wanted to be.

Kate, another woman on our trip, had just called off her wedding. Before the trip, her social media posts about her upcoming wedding made her relationship seem like the perfect fairy tale. She had been with her fiancé for seven years before they decided to get engaged and they had grown through so much together. They had been stepping into their different careers (both what society would label successful) and dreams. But as he traveled more for work and became less flexible to meet her needs, she continued to shift herself to make the relationship work. It took her years before she realized how much she had been focusing on the relationship, so much so that she had ignored her own needs. She barely knew what she really wanted anymore. So, despite all the reasons to go through with the wedding, and all the opinions of everyone, she decided to choose herself (and in the grand scheme of things also her fiancé) and canceled their wedding. Like Farah and myself, this trip was her way of grounding herself back to who she was and discovering herself all over again.

These women's stories are examples of what it means to be beautifully brave. That trip was the beginning of us coming together to heal and stand in our power. If I hadn't said yes, despite my own pride and embarrassment, I would have never known that we all were feeling lost and that there was nothing wrong with me (or any of the other women on the trip). We just needed to find our way back home to ourselves.

We started out as a couple of girls feeling lost, in search of something, and we returned from our two-week trip as brave women committed to never losing ourselves again.

Commit to yourself over and over again, no matter how many times you get lost along the way. The important thing is to always find your way back to you. If you get lost, do things that bring you back to the person you are. And if you don't know what those things are yet, that is okay. Part of discovering yourself again is finding out more about what makes you feel passion in life. Try new things that you've never done before, even if you are scared to do them. Explore different things that you may never have thought you would do or what you've always wanted to do.

Make yourself completely unavailable for things that are not good for you. Go back to those standards we talked about earlier and make sure that you are making them known to those around you, so you never have to compromise yourself. And if there is a misunderstanding of what they are, check in with yourself and with the people you love, and talk it through. Move in love and you will always have space to come back to you.

It can take a while before someone realizes that they need change or how much they have sacrificed themselves for others, but no matter what stage you are in your life, remember that you are always transforming and expanding. You always have time for you. All you have to do is make the commitment to yourself.

**Encourage and support yourself in speaking your truth.**

I love myself
when I give myself
permission to say yes
when I mean yes and
no when I mean no. This
is my life to live and
no one else's.

# 15 WAYS TO NEVER LOSE YOURSELF

**1** **Stand in your power.** Your power is always inside of you ready for you to tap into.

**2** **Move away from avoidance mode.** Oftentimes, we tend to avoid our problems or avoid confronting our fears that we run from them instead of dealing with them head on. By allowing yourself to confront the issues head on and giving the other person an opportunity to change, you are giving yourself and the other person a chance to move forward in love.

**3** **Choose you every time.** Always choose you by allowing yourself to be truthful about what is hurting you and letting someone know when they have crossed a boundary. This will let you know who is meant to go with you on your journey and who isn't.

**4** **Be clear about your standards.** By knowing what you are willing to allow or not allow in your life, you will be able to set boundaries for you to live by. And if anyone compromises those boundaries, you will be able to show up for yourself. Your standards are your compass for how you live and what is allowed to enter into your life.

**5** **Take responsibility for your part.** In any situation where we are struggling, we tend to find a villain in the story and place complete blame on one side. Blaming someone for why a relationship went sour doesn't do anyone any good in healing and growing. By taking responsibility for your role in a situation and only for your role, you are able to give yourself the grace that you deserve and let go of things that are hurtful. You are also allowing the other person to change their ways, and if they don't, then you know that you have to let this person go for your greater well-being.

**6** **Know your triggers.** When we respond from our trigger points, we tend to go back to old negative patterns but when we notice them, we empower ourselves to live a life of healing and understanding. This will help you take responsibility for how you respond to certain situations and what you can do to be better next time.

**7** **Give people the benefit of the doubt.** By choosing to believe the best in others, you are choosing to be open about things before you judge them. This will allow new perspectives, opportunities, and lessons to flow in.

**8** **Do not put someone else above you.** You will never feel worthy enough if you are putting someone up on a pedestal and living from an impossible standard. When you put someone above you, you are silencing yourself. Remember always put yourself first.

**9** **Ask yourself what you contributed to a situation.** By doing this, you are letting yourself take responsibility for only your part in a situation and nothing more. This will keep you from over apologizing. You will also learn from this lesson for the next time a situation like this comes up.

**10** **Give your feelings a voice.** If you keep your feelings inside, you will end up feeling stuck in all that energy. By letting them out, you are clearing out the energy and giving your feelings a safe place to be free.

**11** **Practice ways to clear out any residual energy.** This can look different for everyone and for you it might be a little bit of dancing, screaming, breathwork, or healthy venting.

**12** **Be honest with the people in your life.** Telling the truth is how you show love for yourself and for others.

**13** **Create a safe place for yourself to express your truth.** This allows you to open up, be seen, be heard, and feel safe and secured inside of yourself.

**14** **Stop trying to please other people.** The more you worry about pleasing others, the more you move away from yourself and what you truly want out of life. When you spend more time pleasing yourself, you give yourself the opportunity to learn more about who you are and what your desires are.

**15** **Commit to you.** Become unavailable for things that are not serving you and spend time discovering who you are.

## Homework: Practices That Reflect Your Worth

In what ways can you express yourself, today? How can you reclaim your true self and show up as the woman you were born to be? Before we dive into the following exercise, let me share with you some ideas and rituals that my students and clients love to do. This is just a list to get you started, but have fun with these and create your own as you get more comfortable making self-love a habit. Aim to do one thing a day.

- Cancel plans that you don't want to do to give yourself time for self-care.
- Meditate daily.
- Create gratitude lists.
- Visualize yourself receiving your desires.
- Celebrate yourself even for your smallest wins.
- Drink warm water with lemon in the morning.
- Take yourself on a date.
- Get enough sleep, everyone is different depending on the hours needed. Find yours!
- Host, or go to, dance parties.
- Participate in praise circles.
- Dress up for yourself.
- Bless your food before you eat.
- Buy yourself gifts.
- Go on trips with other women.
- Practice saying "no."
- Set intentions for your day.
- Do more of whatever feels fun for you.

Now that you have taken the time to go over the list, follow this exercise to practice some self-care. Show yourself that you are worth the greatest love of all—the love of you to you.

**Step 1: Gratitude.** Now is the time to thank yourself for all that you are. For even through chaos, a woman treating herself as the goddess she is knows her worth and how to appreciate herself. This can manifest itself in many different ways. You can do this by actively speaking the things you love about yourself or by doing things that let you appreciate your mind, body, and soul. For instance, you can show yourself gratitude by thanking your body and getting a massage after a long week. Choose gratitude practices that ignite something inside of you and make you feel alive.

**Step 2: Pleasure.** A woman in love with herself has fun; she knows that is the point of life. She knows she is worthy of pleasure, that she is worthy of joy. What were the last five things that you experienced that gave you pleasure or that you had so much fun doing? Loving yourself means having fun with yourself. What we think is fun changes, so because you're worth knowing yourself, check in and see what would light you up. What do you need to be adding to your life to be having *a lot* of fun?

Now, make a list of all the things that you think are fun. After you are done with this list, mark next to each the last time you did that thing. Next, schedule one of the things right away and use this to create more of what you love in your life.

**Step 3: Desire.** Desires are not selfish; in fact, it is your birthright to receive. Do not buy into any other story that says something different. Claiming what you want is part of owning your worth. It's your responsibility to stand for yourself and speak those desires into existence. So, this is not just a fun exercise but also a practice you will get *really* good at! The more specific you are, the more the universe will be able to deliver exactly what you asked for. Here are a few examples to get you stated:

- I desire to have a lake house in Austin, with four bedrooms so that I can have friends for vacation, large windows, a dock for a boat, and a gorgeous white kitchen.

- I desire to have financial freedom, to have an abundance of money flowing in and out. I will do what I love and be able to give back to causes I believe in and make a difference in the world.

**Higher Love Level:** Reflect back through your journey and take the time to answer these questions. Once you have your answers, work on the things that need to change. Come back to these questions often.

- What have I been pretending *not* to know?
- Have I been speaking my truth?
- Do I feel lost anywhere inside myself? If yes, in what way?
- What do I need to do for myself?

**You are worthy of self-love and more, so cultivate the goddess in you.**

# I LOVE THE LIFE I HAVE

# *Chapter 7*

# CONNECTING TO YOUR SOUL

**YOUR SOUL ALWAYS** wants to be connected to you. Your soul doesn't care about the fancy house, successful career, or how many social-media followers you have. Your soul cares about the experience of life.

Your soul wants to create with you, feel joy, feel love, feel adventure, feel the experiences that being here on this planet allows it to feel. Only here can you feel what it is like to be human and to feel all emotions. Your soul wants what it wants, and one of the things it calls out for is you.

Your soul cares only about what the fancy house ignites inside you, what the high-profile career creates in you; it wants you to have everything you desire because it wants to experience the joy, gratitude, purpose, and love that you feel when you receive these things. If these material things bring you suffering, fear, jealousy, or feelings of scarcity, you will feel disconnected from your soul. You will always be searching for something, and there will never be enough for you until you reconnect with your soul. Loving yourself is a journey, a relationship that never ends, and part of this journey is a search for yourself that will continue to guide you to a path back to you whenever you need it, back to your soul. . . back home.

> **Loving yourself is a journey, a relationship that never ends. Part of this journey is a search for yourself that will continue to guide you to a path back to you, to your soul back home.**

You must step into or away from many things in order to begin. Some of these things will be toxic to you or will seem big and scary. The imposter syndrome will possibly show up, but you will take the step anyway because you know it's all part of the journey and that the fear isn't real. The big, scary dreams or goals, or whatever it is, are meant for you. When self-doubt shows up, which it will, you can remind yourself, "This isn't truly real. Thank you for trying to help me, but I don't need you to protect me." Once you take the first step, you will begin to build the reference points of remembering that these doubts are just your mind thinking it's keeping you safe. Say thank you to these little doubts and let them know you don't need them to protect you.

Stepping into things that align with your soul will also sometimes mean saying "no" to perfectly great opportunities, places, things, or people because you know it's not the next-level soul joy opportunity for you. And knowing that is your answer. Beginning, not knowing the answer, or just starting new has become such an unwanted experience in society. But it's where the magic is, it's where your soul feels most alive, and it's what has to happen for you to connect to yourself in new and exciting ways.

We live in a world where people want transformation when things have gotten bad, not in a society where we are encouraged to listen to our soul even when things aren't so bad. We want to "get there," but there is no "there." You are here to live out more than getting to one place. You are meant to experience an abundance of everything you wish for. To do that, you must begin somewhere, you must shift, you must embrace yourself even when and if no one else understands it yet. It's business between you and your soul only.

Your soul wants you to do the thing that feels scary. Your soul wants you to expand and trust and believe in yourself. Your soul doesn't want you to settle for okay. It wants you to reach for your highest self, your highest expansion. Just as long as you take the first steps, you're listening to your soul. It will find a way to show you. You don't need to have all the answers, all you need is to listen to your soul's calls and follow the nudges. No one else can tell you what's right or wrong or what you should be doing. What you're doing and who you are have never been done before. There has been no other you. But you aren't alone; your soul is with you and wants to always be connected to you. No one else has gone on this journey before because they aren't you. When you bring more trust and faith to your soul, you will step into who you are.

Society doesn't celebrate you walking away from the "okay" or "good enough." Our society only celebrates "big" achievements. There doesn't have to be a problem for you to begin to go in another direction. You aren't here in this world to just feel all right about life, saying, "I have nothing to complain about, so it's fine." Your soul wants you to feel alive and have the experiences that life has to offer you. You don't have to change direction or make a new decision only when things are visibly failing. What if you chose to shift and walk in another direction just because you knew that the feeling of joy, love, and deep connection was the other way? How different would your life be? The bravery is in walking through fear and walking away from what isn't best for you.

> **If we celebrate ourselves in these brave moments rather than after things worked out, we would influence a new society of women embracing who they are.**

What if we celebrated people for their brave moments in the actual moment? These beautifully brave women would be living a life truly to the fullest, one that is meant only for them, while being honored for their individuality and courageous choices. Our society focuses on the big achievements and checklist goals, and while there is nothing wrong with big achievements, material items, or checklists, imagine how many free and fulfilled souls would be walking around if we honored and celebrated doing what is best for ourselves. We'd be saying no to "good enough" so we can say yes to "incredible."

> **What if you celebrated walking away from a big opportunity that wasn't for you so that you could then walk into something even better? How different would life be?**

Often, things are fine, there's nothing wrong . . . until there is. Until months or years go by and you realize the fire inside of you that wants to live has been told "no" so many times or has been ignored that you are not quite sure what you want anymore. Start to cocreate with that fire now and live a life of joy, fun, and peace; whatever your soul is nudging you to do, do it. All you have to do is take a step toward it and you will be guided to what is next.

Right now, my soul is calling me into a new expansion of my mission. It feels so big and scary, but it also feels like home. When I explain this to people, some think it's funny, or too big; some have thought it's amazing and they can imagine me there. Either point of view really doesn't matter, only mine does for this goal of mine. Though it supports your humanness to be surrounded by those who understand, choosing to be surrounded by them is another form of taking care of yourself. When my ego wakes me up at night to tell me, "Are you sure this will work out? But how do you know, Sarah? They said it just doesn't happen for people like us!" my soul calms me into knowing it will work out and that all I need to do is listen and move with inspired action.

For one of my best friends, Jenna, her soul led her to leave California to move to Texas with her family. She has been like a soul sister to me. She has shown me how much I can trust in sisterhood and know that someone always has my back. I know our friendship will not change, but I am sad she is moving. I want to be able to see her whenever I want. I catch myself doing what society does and thinking, "How can she leave? Her life here is amazing. She doesn't know anyone where she is going!" But that is what I want, not what is best for her. So, I remember why she is leaving: she felt the call to move, there's something there for her in Texas that her soul and the universe know she is meant for. She doesn't know exactly how it's going to be there. It wasn't an easy step to make, but she felt her soul tell her that is where she and her family need to be. And my soul knows that it's her life and her path, and because I love her, I honor that and know something beyond just good is waiting for her there.

Anyone meant for you, anything meant for you, anything that is here to contribute to your highest self, will never leave once you understand that you cannot lose anything that your soul desires. You will lead your life standing in your power and not giving it away to anything outside of you.

For you, maybe your nudge is stepping away from a relationship, changing your career, moving to another place, taking a chance on someone new, or saying "yes" to being beautifully brave. Whatever it is, if you are feeling it in your soul, it's meant for you. If you begin to trust the nudges and choose yourself over the rules and checklists that society says must be met before another step is made, when you throw that out the window, you will live the rest of your life full of love for yourself and joy for what you get to experience. The frequency that you vibe at will attract anything you need and desire. When nothing makes sense, yet it still works out, it will be because you said "yes" and you decided to cocreate with your soul. Once you wake up to your soul and remember it's you, you will never feel alone again. You will know that you aren't alone, and you will feel that deep love and joy inside, because you are on a mission, a journey. You are a gift, and you are creating with the most powerful energy there is. Anything and everything you could ever need is inside of you, it *is* you.

I love myself
when I shift and
evolve to follow my
soul's calling.

However you cocreate these callings, messages, intuitive hits, or whatever you resonate with calling it, your soul is here to take care of yourself. Use the practices in this book so that when you come up against your ego, or external circumstances, or the opinions of others, or your own fear, you will know what to do and those external things won't have as strong of a hold over you. When you empower yourself to listen, trust, take steps, and take care of yourself, you become beautifully brave and continue to be brave no matter what.

It's a brave choice to say, "Some of this doesn't make logical sense, but it makes sense in my heart; it makes sense in my soul." It is a brave choice to decide you're worthy of this care for yourself. Only you can prove to yourself this worth, and only you can decide to believe it. You are worthy of this love, this type of love will feel so deep at times it might be scary, but you know you're brave, you know your way more than enough, and you know you are a gift to this world. You know life is also a gift, and you're here to live it and feel it as your own. You are worthy to be the love of your own life.

In the journey of reconnecting with your soul, you reach a point that your human consciousness is pulled inward toward self-realization. When you are busy saying "yes" to all the things placed on you from external circumstance or opinions and "no" to your own opinion and calling, you're pulled away from yourself. It's when you consciously decide to say "no" and "yes" for you that you begin to be pulled into self-reflection, and it will be easier to feel alignment throughout your inner world. Once this begins, you will notice that you are able to step away from many external opinions, demands, and requests that you had been navigating and allowing into your everyday life.

You will begin to be guided and open to a conscious inner life that is guided by your soul, your desires, and your truth. You may hear people talk about spiritual awakening, and this is the awakening that your soul is calling for! Your consciousness evolves as your soul awakens. We evolve through the heart. This inner love is unlimited and is as infinite as the universe itself. You must be the goddess of your own life, the one who is aware that when self-doubt, worries, desperation, and fear step in, your goddess self will be there to open your heart despite everything.

# YOUR HIGHEST SELF

**KNOWING YOUR HIGHEST** self and being open in your heart is your true nature. Everything else has been junk added from the outside world. Think about our natural reaction to save others when danger appears; it's because that is our truest natural reaction. Somewhere along the way you have felt some magic within yourself; you have felt something powerful, mysterious, loving, and full of light. In today's society, it is very easy to become distant from our highest selves. It can be hard to understand, but when we are aligned with our highest selves, we rise above our conditioned fears, our ego, our limiting beliefs, and our wounds, and only loving ourselves matters. Our highest self is completely free, but it can be blocked or repressed by our ego or our smallness. You are in your smallness when you are living in fear, repressing your feelings, and not following your heart.

**Your highest self is always there: it wants out, it wants to play, it wants to be, it wants to embrace life with you.**

My wish and mission is that wherever you are on your journey, my soul, my heart, and my highest self want to do big things with you in this world. We are connected and my mission is for all of us to move forward and shine in this movement by cocreating a life filled with these practices and insights and by supporting other women up the ladder to their highest self, because doing so will change the world. Each person you lift up and bring with you by sharing your highest, magnetic self will cause a ripple effect so big that the energy and vibrancy around you will shift and you will experience even more love in your inner world. This love and energy will then ripple out to reach further than you will ever truly understand. To embrace your highest self seems like the scariest thing to do because of how powerful it is, yet it is your true nature. Everything else that has kept you from your true nature is not the real you. Uncouple yourself from all the things that were never really you so that you can be who you were meant to be in the first place.

# YOUR SOUL IS THE REAL YOU

**WHEN YOU FEEL** out of alignment, lost, or a deep burning or fire inside to take a different step in your life, become aware of this feeling. Ask the real you what it needs. Feeling "off" is a gift (if you are aware of it) because it's the signal that you are not being or accessing the real you. It's a sign so that you can decide to shift and listen to the real you.

You can decide to notice you feel off and reach for those quick fixes. You can do nothing and continue to feel completely low vibration until the universe hits you in the face and forces you to wake up. Or you can choose to be connected to your highest self, to embrace who you are so that you can have what every human wants—deep, unconditional, unwavering love, the kind of love inside that cannot be explained.

When you acknowledge your soul, you'll begin to hear what it wants, you'll begin to feel those heart strings pull, letting you know it's there, it wants to connect and work together with your heart. The more you leave space to listen to your soul, the more you will feel a surge of love come over you, and your body will fill up with emotions and remembrance. This is your soul's joy and unwavering love for you, acknowledging that you have finally woken up and remembered it. It's a powerful reunion. When you wake up to your desires, you are giving yourself a huge blessing. By making the conscious choice to start honoring and appreciating your soul and to do your very best to stop allowing other things to get in the way of your connection and your purpose, your quality of life and connection to the universe will be life altering in ways that you may have never realized are possible.

I love myself
when I reach for my
highest self.

> **The bravest thing you can do is stay connected to your soul. That connection is the most beautiful gift of all.**

Not everyone will understand it, and people will question it. It's not their life; it's not their soul's purpose to understand yours. People who love you want to keep you safe. They don't want change because it will impact their life and the way they like to do things. One day, because you decided to fully live, they may see that and decide to do the same. That is why choosing yourself is beautifully brave. Standing in your power lets you connect with your soul, show up for the mission, and live each day as if it's the only day that matters.

When you choose to live in the now, what you get in return is unlike anything you could ever imagine—your bravery. Choosing yourself will not only present you with all of life's gifts, but it will also fill you up with a connection so powerful that you will inspire others. You will shift and change the world because you will ignite a power and love so great, you will vibrate at a frequency so high, that you will impact the energy around you. This is all connected to more than we can possibly ever truly understand. We free ourselves when we give love to ourselves, and when we do this, we free others. A world filled with unwavering, praising, unconditional love for self and others is the way of the future.

You can start now by deciding to go on this journey of embracing who you are and loving yourself unconditionally. You can start by placing your hand on your heart, closing your eyes, smiling, and saying, "I know you are here and I love you. Will you stay with me and guide me? How can we go higher? I want to do this life with you."

I love myself
when I unconditionally
embrace who I am.

# 10 WAYS TO CONNECT TO YOUR SOUL

**1** **Step away from things that don't serve you.** Step away from self-doubt. When you choose to continue on your path even though it is big and scary, you are choosing to let go of fear and act in courage. You are listening to what you want and allowing yourself to make your dreams a reality.

**2** **Step into things that align with your soul.** You are meant to experience everything you wish for and more. Your soul wants you to expand and to grow, so move in alignment of your dreams.

**3** **Celebrate the little things.** Every little thing that moves you closer to your soul's desire, no matter how small, is deserving of celebration.

**4** **Shift directions even when everything is going okay.** Move in the direction of joy, and love, move in bravery, even when you don't know where it will lead. Don't wait for things to get bad before making a decision that is for the best of you.

**5** **Listen to your soul.** Your soul will always nudge you wherever you are meant to go next even if you don't know why. When something amazing is waiting for you on the horizon, it is your soul's job to follow suit.

**6** **Take time for self-reflection.** When you self-reflect, you are able to silence external opinions and factors and look within for guidance.

**7** **Release your highest self.** Your highest self is always there, waiting for you to reach for her. Embracing your highest self will cause a ripple effect so big that you will be surrounded by so much love within your inner self.

**8** **Be open in your heart.** Opening your heart is how you open yourself to living a life full of purpose, happiness, and love. Follow your heart and where it leads you.

**9** **Ask yourself what you need.** When you stop allowing other things to get in the way of your purpose, and begin listening to your truest self, you will be able to move toward your soul's calling and living a life full of love.

**10** **Choose to live in the now.** When you decide to live in the now, you are choosing to embrace who you are and to live in bravery. You will foster such a strong connection to your soul that you will impact the world around you.

## Homework: Visualize Your Highest Self

Visualization is a powerful tool. As I've mentioned earlier, this is a great way to visualize what you want to manifest into your life. Use this to connect every part of you and step into your highest self.

**Step 1:** Close your eyes and place your hand on your heart. Breathe into your body, breathe into your heart, and use your breath to carry the energy and light up every part of you, from head to toe. Imagine yourself as the radiant being that you are.

**Step 2:** Call your highest self forth. Imagine her walking through life with a glow of light all around her. Who is surrounding her? What is she doing? Watch her doing whatever it is you desire to be doing and watch her doing it with grace, love, and confidence. Breathe into your heart.

**Step 3:** Take the light that surrounds her and picture it filling you up, starting with your heart, a glow, that moves its way throughout your body. Feel the sensations and imagine yourself going through your day, your life, the world in your power. Once you begin to feel a smile upon your face and tingling in your body, you can begin to close out your visualization by thanking your highest self for being there. Place your hand on your heart filling it with gratitude, touch your face, hug your body and slowly begin to open your eyes. Take this feeling with you throughout the day and come back to it by placing your hands on your heart.

**Higher Love Level:** After you've taken some time to practice this exercise in visualizing your highest self, take time to explore other ways to connect to that power every day. Use these tools to come back to you anytime you need to.

### Other Ways to Access Your Highest Self Daily

Among the power of visualizing your highest self, here are some potent ways you can access your highest self and call her forward. Think of these steps as a starting point. Once you make the following techniques daily habits, you'll be able to create your own unique ways of igniting this power within you.

**Soul writing.** When you write or journal without censoring yourself, you are able to hear from your soul and sort things out that cannot be sorted out the same way in your mind. There is a power in the flow of a pen, and when you do this daily, you give yourself permission to think freely and be uncensored. When you make journaling a habit, you begin to open up the connection to your soul and you train yourself to let thoughts flow without judgment. Soul writing can open up so many doors. You can do this for just 10 minutes a day and it will become something that you look forward to doing with yourself.

**Meditate every day.** You have heard this before, probably dozens of times. Here is why it's important: meditation can be the closest moment you have to God, spirit, your soul, the universe, or whatever you choose to call it. It is a moment that you are completely tapped in, present, open, and available to receive a deep, endless love and an inner peace. Meditation does not need to be complicated, and there is no right or wrong way to do it. Consider giving yourself 5 minutes of silence, prayer, or gratitude every day. In these moments, you connect deeper to your soul.

**Get in tune with nature.** Spend time in nature so that you can begin to recognize the inner knowing your soul is speaking to you. When you decide that you are worthy of this type of love and support for yourself, you will never need to question what is right for you. The gift of connecting to your soul, your highest self, is that you when you get off track you now know how to access it. You know all the ways to get back to you. When you want to deepen your connection to self, go outside. Nature is a gift to us that connects us in energies and frequencies that have us vibrating in love.

**Do something you love.** Doing what you love is what brings you closest to the real you. When you are doing things that you love, you are deeply taking care of yourself and you are connecting with your soul, your true self. You are honoring your gifts and needs, and letting yourself know that you are worthy, that you are important, and that you have decided to embrace yourself and all parts of you. When you are doing the things you love, you feel a love so deep it radiates from the inside out.

**Practice gratitude daily.** You have your assignment for your gratitude board! Refer back to chapter 2. Gratitude is a very high frequency, and in that frequency, you are vibrating at a pure level of abundance, joy, and love. In this frequency, you can manifest your dreams and feel your soul's love. As you use your gratitude board daily, you will begin to see magic happening around you and miracles happening in your life. Gratitude is a connection to your soul, it's honoring and acknowledging the things you have in your life, it's reminding you of the special moments that life brings, and it brings you home to yourself in ways that you may not always understand.

> Always remember that your soul is your guiding force. When you do things from your soul, you will feel a rise of energy within and all around you.

As you go on your own self-love journey, read
the following words to yourself and go on with love.


*In love with myself,*
*as if there is no one else.*


*I'm here to shine,*
*I'm here to be mine.*


*I won't leave my side,*
*I'm ready to rise, because*
*when I love myself,*
*the whole world comes alive.*

# RESOURCES

## Beautifully Brave Extras!

Come join my free private Beautifully Brave Book Readers Facebook community where we will be connecting, supporting you, and building this movement of beautifully brave women loving themselves and uplifting the world, together. There will be daily resources, support, conversation, and of course, celebration!

**VISIT:** www.facebook.com/groups/beautifullybravecommunity

Check out bonus material on self-care and your personal twenty-one-day self-care plan. Come get some custom resources, programs, and bonuses based solely on you through the stars, chakras, and made *for you* self-care.

**VISIT:** girltalknetwork.org

## Contact Information

To hire Sarah as your MC, host or speaker, visit sarahpendrick.com For private coaching, mentorship, or applying to the Together We Empress Mastermind, please contact **admin@girltalkla.org**

## Social Media

**INSTAGRAM:** @sarahpendrick
**FACEBOOK:** https://www.facebook.com/girltalknetwork
**YOUTUBE:** Sarah Pendrick
**TEXT:** 310-340-2896

It feels like a dream come true to be writing my own acknowledgment section for my book. I want to first acknowledge and thank you for saying "yes" to yourself and picking up this book, making my vision for you and women everywhere possible. I'd like to thank **my soul mate**, **my husband Josh**. You have shown me a safe place that I never knew was possible and an everlasting home that I cannot begin to put into words. You are my king, my best friend, and my family. I found and chose you after I began my journey of loving me, and ever since then, you have supported me in every single thing that I do. I am grateful for you beyond words for the life we continue to build together, and I am grateful to God for bringing you to me. You are my soulmate in every life and my home. **To my parents**: I love you both endlessly. **Dad**, at every point in my life, I have always known that if I was in trouble and needed you to be somewhere that you would stop at nothing to get there. Our relationship has been a great teacher to me. I wish for you the peace and joy you deserve, and I am forever grateful to know how much you love me. **Mom**, thank you for always believing in me. Thank you for your openness and support. You are powerful and have taught me many things throughout my life, including the confidence I carry to know I can achieve

anything. I know we have had many lifetimes together. Thank you being my mother and for everything you do. **To my brothers**, **Adam**, **Chris**, **and Michael**: I love you all more than you could ever know. My heart feels you always. **To my Nana**: we have always shared a very special bond and I carry you with me wherever I go. You are a very inspiring and strong woman and you filled many of my childhood memories with love and joy. **To my godmother**, **Donna Murphy**: I am so grateful to have you in my life. Your support means the world to me and you have cheered me on like no other. **To my soul sisters**: Jenna, Natalie Jill, Sarah Stewart, Natalie Ellis, Danielle, Ashley, Gina, and Dr. Judy Ho, your friendship means the world to me, we have a deep sisterhood and I am beyond grateful for your support—not only in my life but how much you showed up through this book process and supported me with anything I needed. **To my Los Angeles soul sisters**: you all know who you are, our group and love for each other is so special, truly healing sisterhood all over the world. **To my childhood friends**, I love you so much, we grew up together and I am so grateful that we have this strong bond throughout our lives, it's special and it's rare. Jamie, Beth, Jilly, Arielle, Nicole, Bri, Karina, and so many more.

**To my family:** my aunts, uncles, cousins, there are so many of us and you have taught me life lessons, loyalty, and no matter what has ever happened I know that I can always call on you. Thank you for believing in me and cheering me on. **To my amazing editor, Keyla Pizarro-Hernández**, and **publisher, Rage Kindelsperger**. I adore both of you and feel so lucky to work with you and create magic for women. I wished to work with editors who not only believed in me but who also shared the same wishes, dreams, and love for others. This experience has been one I will never forget, and I am so grateful that every step of the way has been like a dream. Keyla, your encouragement, talent, and dedication have made such a difference in this process. Rage, from the beginning you believed in this; your spirit, talent, and energy are such a gift to this world. **To all of my clients, partners, and GirlTalk Community**, you are my why and my inspiration. I am so humbled by your dedication and your love. I am honored to be a part of your journey and blown away daily by your commitment and the community we have built together. I couldn't do any of this without you and I love you from my whole heart. **To my GirlTalk Festival Attendees**, you make the world go round and I look forward to being with you every year, together we create a ripple effect with the energy and transformation that takes place on that stage, in that room and throughout our yearly weekend together. **To my Women Leader's Mastermind "Together We Empress" group**: together we are truly changing the world and giving women the fullest permission to live a life in love with themselves. Thank you for allowing me to create this container and lead you, I am so incredibly grateful and honored to expand and uplevel the planet with you. You are changing the way women do business, take care of themselves and connect. This is a new way, a better way, and a way that is natural inside of us. Cheers to your everlasting abundance and success! I love you and I am honored to do this work with you. This is one of my most favorite programs and creations, thank you for being a part of it. **To my SP and GirlTalk teams**, I couldn't do this without you. I am grateful for you each and every day. **To my program team and writing team, Sarah Fields**, thank you for always being up for anything and there to support this book and our mission. Thank you **Kirsten Trammell**, thank you for your feedback, support, and positivity through these chapters and in our projects.

# REFERENCES

Bush, C. R., Bush, J. P., & Jennings, J. (1988). Effects of Jealousy Threats on Relationship Perceptions and Emotions. *Journal of Social and Personal Relationships,* 5(3), 285–303. https://doi.org/10.1177/0265407588053002.

Chapman, G. D., & Green, J. (2017). *The 5 love languages: The secret to love that lasts.* Chicago: Northfield Publishing.

Cole, A. (2016, June 28). Does Your Body Really Refresh Itself Every 7 Years? Retrieved November 11, 2020, from https://www.npr.org/sections/health-shots/2016/06/28/483732115/how-old-is-your-body-really.

Dwelling on negative events biggest cause of stress - University of Liverpool News. (2014, June 17). Retrieved November 11, 2020, from https://news.liverpool.ac.uk/2013/10/17/dwelling-on-negative-events-biggest-cause-of-stress/

Fetus to Mom: You're Stressing Me Out! (n.d.). Retrieved November 13, 2020, from https://www.webmd.com/baby/features/fetal-stress

Leknes, S., Bastian, B. The Benefits of Pain. Rev.Phil.Psych. 5, 57–70 (2014). https://doi.org/10.1007/s13164-014-0178-3.

Liggett, D. R., & Hamada, S. (1993). Enhancing the visualization of gymnasts. *The American Journal of Clinical Hypnosis*, 35(3), 190–197. https://doi.org/10.1080/00029157.1993.10403003.

Mullen, P. E., & Martin, J. (1994). Jealousy: a community study. *The British Journal of Psychiatry : The Journal of Mental Science*, 164(1), 35–43. https://doi.org/10.1192/bjp.164.1.35.

The limbic system. (2019, January 24). Retrieved November 11, 2020, from https://qbi.uq.edu.au/brain/brain-anatomy/limbic-system.

Robinson Ph.D, B. (2020, April 26). The 90-Second Rule That Builds Self-Control. Retrieved November 13, 2020, from https://www.psychologytoday.com/intl/blog/the-right-mindset/202004/the-90-second-rule-builds-self-control?amp.

Social Comparison Theory. (n.d.). Retrieved November 11, 2020, from https://www.psychologytoday.com/us/basics/social-comparison-theory.

Vinney, C. (n.d.). What's the Difference Between Eudaimonic and Hedonic Happiness? Retrieved November 11, 2020, from https://www.thoughtco.com/eudaimonic-and-hedonic-happiness-4783750.